Atlas of Inflammatory Bowel Disease-Associated Intestinal Cancer

Toshiyuki Matsui • Akinori Iwashita
Takayuki Matsumoto • Takashi Hisabe
Kitaro Futami • Hiroshi Tanabe
Editors

Atlas of Inflammatory Bowel Disease-Associated Intestinal Cancer

Examining the Macroscopic Images of Small and Large Intestine

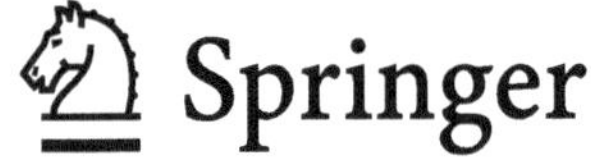

Editors
Toshiyuki Matsui
Fukuoka University
Fukuoka, Japan

Akinori Iwashita
Fukuoka University
Fukuoka, Japan

Takayuki Matsumoto
Department of Internal Medicine
Iwate Medical University
Iwate, Japan

Takashi Hisabe
Department of Gastroenterology
Fukuoka University Chikushi Hospital
Chikushino, Japan

Kitaro Futami
Center for Clinical Medical Research (Surgery)
Fukuoka University Chikushi Hospital
Chikushino, Japan

Hiroshi Tanabe
Department of Pathology
Fukuoka University Chikushi Hospital
Chikushino, Japan

ISBN 978-981-19-3415-5 ISBN 978-981-19-3413-1 (eBook)
https://doi.org/10.1007/978-981-19-3413-1

The translation was done with the help of artificial intelligence (machine translation by the service DeepL.com). A subsequent human revision was done primarily in terms of content.
Translation from the Japanese language edition: "Enshosei Cho Shikkan Kanren Cho Gan Atlas" by Toshiyuki Matsui et al., © Toshiyuki Matsui 2021. Published by CBR Publishers Inc.. All Rights Reserved.

This Springer imprint is published by the registered company Springer Nature Singapore Pte Ltd.
The registered company address is: 152 Beach Road, #21-01/04 Gateway East, Singapore 189721, Singapore

Preface

Inflammatory bowel disease (IBD)-associated cancers have increased significantly and are no longer rare. For endoscopist, therefore, it has become necessary to deal with them in routine diagnosis. In other words, knowledge in this field should be considered essential. Research papers are also increasing. Recently, a systematic review and meta-analysis of prognostic factors for IBD-associated bowel cancer was published in Gastroenterology (2020). 18 factors were identified, and more than 10,000 IBD-associated cancer papers were cited in the search. They narrowed down the list to 164 papers for analysis. Research on IBD-associated cancers has been active for 40 years. In particular, research on surveillance has been increasing rapidly. However, progress in endoscopic diagnosis has been slow. There have been few major developments since the SCENIC consensus published in 2015, which is described in this book. Endoscopic equipment has increased, but there has been no breakthrough in diagnostic studies. The reason for this may be that this disease is relatively rare and few endoscopists have experienced many actual cases. Therefore, we believe that it is truly meaningful to gather many cases in one place and systematically display them.

There is also confusion regarding pathological diagnosis. In Europe and the United States, Riddell's classification (1983) is used, and there has been no significant change since then. In Japan, on the other hand, the classification of the Research Group for Intractable Intestinal Disorders of Specified Diseases of the Ministry of Health, Labour and Welfare (1994) is used. Although it is possible to compare them, it is difficult to use them in English papers. In this book, the diagnosis is developed in accordance with the diagnosis of intestinal tumors, and the term "dysplastic epithelium" is used when it is difficult to determine whether a lesion is neoplastic or inflammatory. In addition, lesions with dysplasia alone, for which the diagnostic criteria are ambiguous, are not included. Another feature of this book is the careful pathological diagnosis. In our institution, we have many surgical cases of IBD, and all resected specimens are divided and several hundred step section specimens are prepared. The basic attitude of Professor Iwashita and Dr. Tanabe is strongly reflected in this book.

This book is characterized by the contrast between the endoscopic image and the pathological construct. Because these conversations and discussions are routinely working between pathologists and endoscopists. The reason why lesions are difficult to see and identify is explained so that the reader can understand them clearly. A feature of this book is the atlas of each case, in which UC-associated cancer and CD-associated cancer are described separately. CD-associated cancers are often more difficult to diagnose than UC-associated cancers, partly because endoscopes are unable to reach the lesion site due to intestinal stenosis, and partly because the affected area is often perianal or ileal region where mucosal inflammation is severe and destructive changes are obvious. The initial lesions are located at the margins of the ulcer and have a morphology similar to type III cancer, so the definite diagnosis must rely on postoperative search. "Invisible" is one of the keywords of this book, and we have tried to prove that the lesions are truly invisible. We hope that you will understand through our presentation.

The editor of this book, Professor Takayuki Matsumoto, is one of the committee members who participated in the SCENIC consensus and is a leading expert in this field. He participated in both the general and specific sections. Prof. Akinori Iwashita is a leading expert in gastrointestinal tumor pathology and inflammatory bowel disease pathology. Dr. Iwashita and Dr. Hiroshi Tanabe participated in the overall pathology review and case presentation. Prof. Kitaro Futami contributed to this article with a special focus on CD-associated cancer. He has focused on perianal carcinogenesis, which is unique in Japan and has carried out a lot of surveillance. He will present his results and data in the review section. Associate Professor Takashi Hisabe has been analyzing UC-associated cancers for many years. Based on his studies if the lesion had been invisible by surveillance endoscopy 2 years ago, the examining physician would not have been responsible, but if a biopsy had been performed, a different conclusion might have been reached. In the case of UC-associated cancers that are ultimately found to be advanced, there is a high probability that the lesion would have been identified on surveillance 2 years earlier, and it may be possible to discuss the concept of interval cancer again and recommend that aggressive biopsy should be incorporated for early diagnosis during surveillance.

This book is intended for all those who are involved in endoscopic surveillance. We are confident that some of the presented cases will be of interest to even the most experienced endoscopist.

Chikushino, Fukuoka, Japan Toshiyuki Matsui

May 5, 2021

Contents

Contributors

Makoto Eizuka Department of Molecular Diagnostic Pathology, Iwate Medical University, Iwate, Japan

Department of Gastroenterology, Iwate Medical University, Iwate, Japan

Minako Fujiwara Department of Pathology, National Hospital Organization Kyushu Medical Center, Fukuoka, Japan

Kitaro Futami Center for Clinical Medical Research (Surgery), Fukuoka University Chikushi Hospital, Chikushino, Japan

Takashi Hisabe Department of Gastroenterology, Fukuoka University Chikushi Hospital, Chikushino, Japan

Koji Ikegami Department of Medicine and Clinical Science, Graduate School of Medical Sciences, Kyushu University, Fukuoka, Japan

Akinori Iwashita Fukuoka University, Fukuoka, Japan

Keisuke Kawasaki Department of Gastroenterology, Iwate Medical University, Iwate, Japan

Department of Medicine and Clinical Science, Graduate School of Medical Sciences, Kyushu University, Fukuoka, Japan

Toshiyuki Matsui Fukuoka University, Fukuoka, Japan

Takayuki Matsumoto Department of Gastroenterology, Iwate Medical University, Iwate, Japan

Tamotsu Sugai Department of Molecular Diagnostic Pathology, Iwate Medical University, Iwate, Japan

Hiroshi Tanabe Department of Pathology, Fukuoka University Chikushi Hospital, Chikushino, Japan

Part I

Bowel Cancer Associated with IBD: Overview

Intestinal Cancer Associated with IBD: Aim and Structure of This Book

Toshiyuki Matsui

1 Background

Inflammatory bowel disease (IBD)-associated intestinal cancer has been diagnosed and treated mainly in Europe and the United States. In Japan, IBD-associated colorectal cancer (CRC) has been increasing, and although ulcerative colitis (UC) surgery itself has been decreasing, CRC has been reported to account for a large proportion (34.8%) of the reasons for colorectal resection surgery [1], suggesting that countermeasures are urgently needed. Since CRC diagnosis in advanced cancer does not improve the prognosis, efficient surveillance endoscopy methodologies have been discussed to pick up early-stage cancer. In this context, the Japanese classification of early-stage colorectal cancer has been used as the Paris classification, which is a universal gross classification of superficial CRC [2]. Based on this classification, progress has been made in endoscopic diagnosis and techniques for UC-related cancers, and dye method and target biopsy is becoming the basic technique [3, 4]. However, there is a need for a more reliable diagnosis method. The reason for this is that there is an opportunity to diagnose smaller dysplasia or early-stage cancer and to seek endoscopic treatment. However, these advances have not progressed as expected because of the current limitations of endoscopic diagnostic capability and pathological diagnosis.

In Crohn's disease (CD), not only CRC but also small bowel cancer (SBC) is increasingly being detected clinically. The increase in the number of diagnosed cases is comparable to the increase in the number of UC cases [5]. The number of cases of carcinogenesis in CD is not as large as that in UC. In a recent meta-analysis of CD-related cancer cases by Uchino et al., the prevalence of colorectal cancer (CRC) was estimated to be 0.77% in CD cases and 0.23% in small bowel cancer (SBC) cases [5]. In Japan, the standardized incidence ratio (SIR) of CRC in CD is the same as that in Europe and the United States (SIR; 2.08 worldwide, 1.1–2.2 in Europe and the United States, and 3.2–5.8 in Japan). Furthermore, it has been pointed out that in Japan and Asia, many cases of CD carcinogenesis are located in the anorectal region (63% on the left side in Europe and the United States and 84% on the left side in Asia) [5]. Considering this tendency, original surveillance in Japan is being sought. Furthermore, CRC is often detected in advanced cancer, and the prognosis for life after surgery is not good. The risk factors for CRC in CD identified in Japan are as follows: (1) female, (2) history of surgery, (3) history of disease for more than 20 years, (4) onset at age 25 years or younger, (5) small and large intestine type, and (6) presence of anorectal lesions [6]. According to Yasukawa, the mortality rate due to CRC in CD cases is high, and cancer accounts for 10–15% of disease-specific mortality [7]. On the other hand, many European and American general population statistics report that the incidence of CRC in patients with IBD is decreasing year by year, and the decrease is particularly marked in UC [8, 9]. The reason for this is thought to be that surveillance is conducted efficiently or that therapeutic agents such as biologics have advanced and can suppress inflammation for a long time. However, in a recent report by King in the UK, the number of IBD patients is increasing in the UK, and CRC is increasing in UC [10]. In any case, an understanding of the current situation is probably an important step in dealing with the occurrence of CRC.

T. Matsui (✉)
Fukuoka University, Fukuoka, Japan
e-mail: matsui@fukuoka-u.ac.jp

T. Matsui et al. (eds.), *Atlas of Inflammatory Bowel Disease-Associated Intestinal Cancer*,
https://doi.org/10.1007/978-981-19-3413-1_1

2 Aim and Structure of This Book

The issues in this book are summarized in the following few points;

2.1 To understand the clinical and pathological picture of IBD-associated intestinal cancer

The primary purpose of this atlas is to contrast endoscopic images of IBD carcinogenesis cases with resected intestinal mucosal gross and histological images. There have been only a few atlases that present gross images of IBD-related cancers, such as Matsumoto's in 2006 and Soetikno's in 2014 [11, 12]. In particular, there have been few images of CD-associated cancers. Furthermore, there are no studies comparing UC and CD carcinogenesis cases. There have also been few presentations of diagnosed cases of anorectal cancer, which has been increasing in our country.

In addition, many IBD-associated cancers are superficial lesions that are difficult to diagnose. The presence of inflammatory changes in the surrounding area makes diagnosis even more difficult. Even in the United States and Europe, it has been pointed out that there is a limit to the number of elevated lesions that can be considered as the main lesion. Jaramillo et al. reported that the morphology of endoscopically detected tumors (high-grade dysplasia or low-grade dysplasia) in UC was flat in 67% of cases [13]. Sugimoto classified the endoscopic morphology of UC-related high-grade dysplasia or early-stage cancer cases according to the SCENIC consensus [14]. Sugimoto classified the endoscopic morphology of 39 cases of atypical lesions corresponding to early-stage cancer, of which 64% were elevated, 48.7% were superficially elevated, 30.8% were flat, and 5.1% were depressed. In other words, the majority of the gross images were superficial or non-polypoid in shape. In addition, when there is inflammation around the lesion, it is difficult to see the reddening, which is an opportunity to detect the lesion, and the surrounding border becomes less distinct (46% distinct border lesion vs. 54% indistinct border) [14]. Thus, the high prevalence of superficial cancers makes detection of lesions difficult, and IBD-associated cancers are frequently missed.

UC has been considered to have a high number of missed lesions. In Wang's study, which precisely estimated the proportion of missed lesions, it was estimated to be 15% in CD and 16% in UC, whereas it was only 5.8% in non-IBD patients [15]. According to Wang, the proportion of interval cancers is three times higher in CRC patients with IBD than in those with normal CRC. According to Sanduleanu and Rutter [16], the definition of interval cancer is CRC detected by surveillance after initial negative surveillance endoscopy. Based on 40 years of UC surveillance follow-up at St Mark's Hospital the study found that more than half of CRCs corresponded to interval cancer. In the last decade, a gradual downward trend in the proportion of patients with interval cancer has been noted [17]. This definition does not include cases of inappropriate surveillance (inadequate testing, inappropriate intervals between tests). (1) incomplete resection, and (2) suboptimal surveillance. This suggests that the conventional surveillance method of endoscopy plus random biopsy may have limitations. Therefore, it is important for endoscopists to increase their awareness of the morphology of CRC lesions, to become proficient in examination, and to perform appropriate biopsies [16].

2.2 Definition of gross image of IBD-associated cancer; depending on endoscopic superficial images or on combination of endoscopic image and pathological invasion

The mucosal borders of IBD-associated cancers are often difficult to identify. Surrounding dysplasia and very well differentiated carcinoma also make the boundary with noncancerous areas difficult to understand. The visual type has been determined mainly by endoscopic images. Is the definition of dysplasia or cancer reliable? How do we determine the gross type of cancer when the borders are difficult to discern? Is it determined by endoscopic findings alone or by taking into account histopathological findings? Multiple lesions should be easier to detect if the lesions are at least fully circumscribed. In this article, we will discuss these opinions on the gross type of lesion by presenting a case.

2.3 Construction of clinical findings necessary for rational surveillance

It would be good to discuss which findings are useful for the early detection of cancer. In addition, it would be good if we could combine the methods according to the risk that the patient has and link them to an algorithm. The mainstream opinion is that chromoendoscopy + target biopsy is superior to white light + random biopsy for endoscopic techniques, but it would be good if a better method could be found. It is desirable to construct a rational diagnostic process for clinicians in consideration of the above issues.

2.4 The pathological differentiation between sporadic and IBD-related cancers should also be presented and considered

In our institution, we have a basic stance of preparing whole sections of resected specimens for pathological analysis in all cases of IBD surgery, and the results of our studies have been accumulated in conjunction with the increase in IBD-associated cancers. Therefore, four of my colleagues and I planned this book to solve the problem by comparing endoscopic and pathological images using the gross image of the resected specimen as the basic image.

In this book, four review articles are placed at the beginning. (1) Endoscopic diagnosis of UC carcinogenesis based on the SCENIC consensus (site, diagnostic occasion, precise imaging, and surveillance procedures), (2) Characteristics of CD carcinogenesis; carcinogenic sites (small intestine, colon, rectum, and anal canal), gross features, and differences from UC-related cancers, (3) pathological cases of UC carcinogenesis and CD carcinogenesis and the differences between them, and (4) the retrospective developmental course of UC carcinogenesis. The reason for this was to analyze how localized findings should be taken by analyzing the preceding endoscopic images in cases that appeared to be interval carcinoma in the course of consecutive surveillance. Some of them were published as endoscopic images of interval carcinoma, which can be used to estimate the growth rate [18, 19]. We believe that this analysis may contribute to the diagnosis of cancer at an earlier stage and provide insight into the speed of cancer progression. Although it involves subjective judgment, it is often possible to recognize a preceding lesion in the rectosigmoid colon, which is easy to identify.

Next, in the atlas section, actual cases of UC carcinogenesis were presented, divided into early-stage and advanced cancers. Finally, CD carcinoma cases were divided into small bowel cancer, colon cancer, rectal cancer, and anal canal cancer. In all cases, the resected specimens were properly obtained from the patients. Cases with solely dysplasia were not included in this presentation. As is well known, the histological diagnosis of dysplasia is not uniform internationally, and it is also difficult to distinguish between low and high atypia, so it is better to describe dysplasia as neoplasia. The pathological diagnosis in this book distinguishes between cancer and non-cancerous conditions; the term dysplastic epithelium is used when neoplasia cannot be diagnosed.

Please read this document with an understanding of the above positions.

References

1. Uchino M, Ikeuchi H, Hata K, et al. Changes in the rate of and trends in colectomy for ulcerative colitis during the era of biologics and calcineurin inhibitors based on a Japanese nationwide cohorts survey. Surg Today. 2019;49:1066–73.
2. The Paris endoscopic classification of superficial neoplastic lesions: esophagus, stomach, and colon: November 30 to December 1, 2002. Gastrointest Endosc. 2003;58(6 Suppl):S3–43.
3. Laine L, Kaltenbach T, Barkun A, et al. SCENIC international consensus statement on surveillance and management of dysplasia in inflammatory bowel disease. Gastrointest Endosc. 2015;81:489–501.
4. Watanabe T, Ajioka Y, Mitsuyama K, et al. Comparison of targeted vs random biopsies for surveillance of ulcerative colitis-associated colorectal cancer. Gastroenterology. 2016;151(6):1122–30.
5. Uchino M, Ikeuchi H, Hata K, et al. Intestinal cancer in patients with Crohn's disease: a systematic review and meta-analysis. J Gastroenterol Hepatol. 2020;35:1–8.
6. Yano Y, Matsui T, Hirai F, et al. Cancer risk in Japanese Crohn's disease patients: investigation of the standardized incidence ratio. J Gastroenterol Hepatol. 2013;28:1300–5.
7. Yasukawa S, Matsui T, Yano Y, et al. Crohn's disease-specific mortality: a 30-year cohort study at a tertiary referral center in Japan. J Gastroenterol. 2019;54(1):42–52.
8. Jess T, Simonsen J, Jørgensen KT, et al. Decreasing risk of colorectal cancer in patients with inflammatory bowel disease over 30 years. Gastroenterology. 2012;143:375–81.
9. Castaño-Milla C, Chaparro M, Gisbert JP. Systematic review with meta-analysis: the declining risk of colorectal cancer in ulcerative colitis. Aliment Pharmacol Ther. 2014;39(7):645–59.
10. King D, Reulen RC, Thomas T, et al. Changing patterns in the epidemiology and outcomes of inflammatory bowel disease in the United Kingdom: 2000-2018. Aliment Pharmacol Ther. 2020;51(10):922–34. https://doi.org/10.1111/apt.15701.
11. Matsumoto T, Iwao Y, Igarashi M, et al. Endoscopic and chromoendoscopic atlas featuring dysplastic lesions in surveillance colonoscopy for patients with long-standing ulcerative colitis. Inflamm Bowel Dis. 2006;14:259–64.
12. Soetikno R, Sanduleanu S, Kaltenbach T. An atlas of nonpolypoid colorectal neoplasms in inflammatory bowel disease. Gastrointest Endosc Clin N Am. 2014;24:483–520.
13. Jaramillo E, Watanabe M, Befrits R, et al. Small, flat colorectal neoplasias in long-standing ulcerative colitis detected by high-resolution electronic video endoscopy. Gastrointest Endosc. 1996;44(1):15–22.
14. Sugimoto S, Naganuma M, Iwao Y, et al. Endoscopic morphologic features of ulcerative colitis-associated dysplasia classified according to the SCENIC consensus statement. Gastrointest Endosc. 2017;85(3):639–46.
15. Wang YR, Cangemi JR, Loftus EV Jr, Picco MF. Rate of early/missed colorectal cancers after colonoscopy in older patients with or without inflammatory bowel disease in the United States. Am J Gastroenterol. 2013;108:444–9.
16. Sanduleanu S, Rutter MD. Interval colorectal cancers in inflammatory bowel disease: the grim statistics and true stories. Gastrointest Endosc Clin N Am. 2014;24(3):337–48.
17. Choi CH, Rutter MD, Askari A, et al. Forty-year analysis of the colonoscopic surveillance program for neoplasia in ulcerative colitis: an updated overview. Am J Gastroenterol. 2015;110(7):1022–34.
18. Yamasaki K, Matsui T, Hisabe T, et al. Retrospective analysis of the growth speed of 54 lesions of colitis-associated colorectal neoplasia. Anticancer Res. 2016;36(7):3731–40.
19. Hisabe T, Matsui T, Yamasaki K, et al. Possible earlier diagnosis of ulcerative colitis-associated neoplasia: a retrospective analysis of interval cases during surveillance. J Clin Med. 2021;10:1927. https://doi.org/10.3390/jcm10091927.

Endoscopic Diagnosis of Neoplastic Lesions in Inflammatory Bowel Disease

Takayuki Matsumoto

1 Introduction

It is well known that inflammatory bowel disease is a high-risk group for colorectal cancer. In particular, the cumulative incidence of colorectal cancer associated with ulcerative colitis (UC) has been shown to increase to about 10% by 25 years after the initial diagnosis of UC. Furthermore, the number of patients with UC is increasing in Japan, and it is predicted that the frequency of UC-associated neoplastic lesions (UCAN) will increase in the future. In this book, we describe the endoscopic diagnosis of UCAN in Surveillance for Colorectal Endoscopic Neoplasia Detection and Management in Inflammatory Bowel Disease Patients International Consensus Statement (SCENIC) and Frankfurt Advanced Chromoendoscopic Ibd Lesions (FACILE), and discuss the problems of endoscopic diagnosis of UCAN. I would like to consider the problems of endoscopic diagnosis of UCAN.

2 Surveillance Endoscopy in UC

The risk factors for UCAN are known to include the onset of UC at a young age, long-term and extensive morbidity, chronic persistent inflammation, and complications of primary sclerosing cholangitis [1]. (1) On the other hand, although UCAN was traditionally thought to occur in the deep colon in Europe and the United States, it has recently been shown to occur in the distal colon, i.e., the rectum and sigmoid colon [2].

Since the 1980s, surveillance colonoscopy has been recommended for the early detection of UCAN. At that time, it was difficult to diagnose even the presence of UCAN, and therefore in addition to biopsies from lesions suspected of having UCAN (target biopsy), it was recommended to obtain biopsied tissue from apparently nontumor flat mucosa (random biopsy) [1]. (1) Since then, although endoscopic equipment represented by image-enhanced endoscopes has advanced dramatically, there has been no consensus on specific techniques for the diagnosis of UCAN or on the treatment of discovered lesions.

3 SCENIC

3.1 Creation Method

SCENIC was held in 2014 as an international consensus meeting on SC and tumor therapies [3, 4]. For this international meeting, 10 clinical questions (CQs) and their systematic reviews were prepared in advance. Based on these, statements were prepared and voted on in two meetings.

On the other hand, a preliminary meeting was held by the members in charge of terminology to discuss the dye endoscopy method, differentiation between adenoma and dysplasia, and the UCAN gross classification method and its description. In the end, the Paris International Classification [5] was adopted for the gross classification in accordance with the Japanese Colorectal Cancer Code of Practice, and lesions detected only by random biopsy were described as nonvisible lesions. No consensus was reached on the distinction between adenoma and dysplasia.

3.2 Main Statements

1. "For surveillance endoscopy, dye endoscopy is recommended over white-light endoscopy (85% agreement, strong recommendation, moderate level of evidence)."

   The results of the meta-analysis showed that the diagnostic rate of UCAN in target biopsy was 7.5% for white light and 14.1% for dye endoscopy. This result led to the

T. Matsumoto (✉)
Department of Gastroenterology, Iwate Medical University, Iwate, Japan
e-mail: tmatsumo@iwate-med.ac.jp

T. Matsui et al. (eds.), *Atlas of Inflammatory Bowel Disease-Associated Intestinal Cancer*,
https://doi.org/10.1007/978-981-19-3413-1_2

adoption of the above statement with a relatively high agreement rate and a moderate level of evidence. A subsequently reported meta-analysis also proved the superiority of dye endoscopy [6].

2. "NBI endoscopy cannot be recommended as an alternative to dye endoscopy in surveillance endoscopy (90% agreement, weak recommendation, moderate level of evidence)."

   The detection rate of UCAN was higher with dye endoscopy than with NBI endoscopy, but the examination time for dye endoscopy was significantly longer. Therefore, the above statement was adopted. Subsequently, a study using second-generation NBI confirmed its non-inferiority to dye endoscopy [7]. In addition to NBI, LCI, BLI, and endocytoscopy have been reported one after another to be useful in diagnosing the presence of UCAN. The diagnosis of UCAN by image-enhanced endoscopy is discussed in the next section, FACILE, and it will be necessary to transmit clinical data from Japan to the world in this area.

3. "After complete endoscopic resection of endoscopically resectable neoplastic lesions, continued surveillance by endoscopy is recommended over colorectal resection" (elevated lesions; 100% agreement, strong recommendation, low level of evidence. Flat lesions; 80% agreement, weak recommendation, low level of evidence)

   This was a CQ that fundamentally changed the treatment of UCAN. This statement was adopted because the incidence of UCAN was acceptable in a meta-analysis of follow-up cases after endoscopic resection for raised UCAN. However, this statement does not define "endoscopically resectable" lesions, nor does it consider criteria such as "complete" or "incomplete" resection, extent, depth, histology, or differentiation. In a meta-analysis of 14 papers subsequently reported, the cumulative incidence of colorectal cancer in UC patients treated with endoscopic therapy was 2/1000 person-years, which was lower than the incidence of colorectal cancer in UC patients (14/1000 person-years) [8].

4. "Referral to an inflammatory bowel disease specialist with expertise in dye endoscopy is recommended for the diagnosis and treatment of endoscopically unrecognizable neoplastic lesions (100% agreement, weak recommendation, low level of evidence)."

   This section deals with UCANs that are positive on random biopsy. UCANs detected by random biopsy alone account for about 10% of all UCANs, and it is clearly stated that these lesions should be retested with endoscopic treatment in mind. On the other hand, the pros and cons of random biopsy were discussed in SCENIC, but no definite conclusion was reached. This was due to the fact that there was no evidence for random biopsy, and the discussion ended in empiricism. The results of conflicting clinical studies have been reported since then [9, 10], and it is expected that this issue will continue to be discussed in the future.

3.3 Impact of SCENIC

Dysplasia-associated lesion or mass (DALM), which was proposed in the 1980s, is defined as "a grossly elevated lesion histologically consistent with dysplasia" and has been used as an indicator for colorectal resection because DALM-positive cases are frequently accompanied by invasive cancer in other parts of the colon. Since then, DALM has been used as a marker for colorectal resection [11]. Subsequently, DALM came to be used as a general term for elevated UCAN. However, after the widespread use of SCENIC, Riddell et al. recommended avoiding the use of "DALM" and describing it according to the gross classification of SCENIC, because it is difficult to differentiate adenoma from dysplasia in UC [12].

On the other hand, recommendations and guidelines for surveillance endoscopy for UC reported in Europe and the United States in the past did not include any mention of endoscopic treatment, whereas endoscopic treatment for UCAN has been specified as an option in patient management guidelines since SCENIC [2].

4 FACILE [12]

In SCENIC, dye endoscopy was confirmed to be the basic technique for surveillance endoscopy. However, image-enhanced endoscopy is currently the main method of observation in the treatment of colorectal cancer. Therefore, an attempt to search for findings characteristic of UCAN by image-enhanced endoscopic observation such as NBI, i-SCAN, and FICE was made at the international meeting of FACILE. Specifically, the study included UCAN and non-neoplastic lesions observed by the participants using conventional, dye, and image-enhanced endoscopy. Of these lesions, endoscopic findings in lesions outside of their own institution were independently determined, and findings that were specific to neoplastic lesions and had a high rate of agreement among endoscopists were statistically extracted.

One actual example is shown in Fig. 1. The items examined were the gross type (according to the SCENIC classification), the presence or absence of ulceration within the presumed lesion and in the surrounding mucosa, the boundaries of the lesion, color tone, microsurface structure, and microvascular structure. As a result, gross type (odds ratio of surface type: 11.6), irregular microvascular structure (5.1), fine surface structure (3.2), and absence of ulceration within

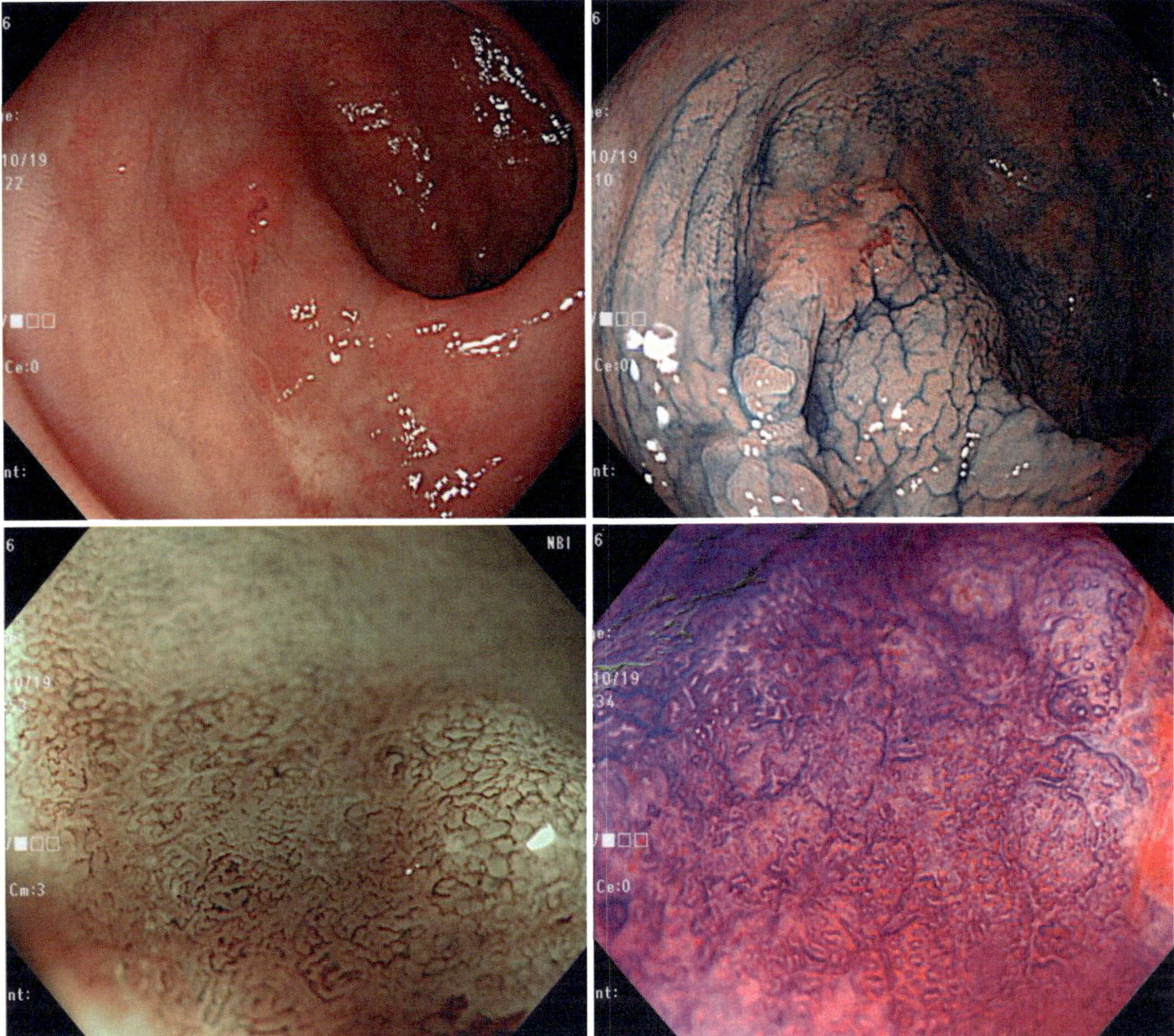

Fig. 1 Example of UCAN with findings judged according to FACILE. The lesion was judged by the author to be flat and depressed, no ulceration in or on the surrounding mucosa, almost the same color tone as the surrounding mucosa, clear borders, irregular microsurface structure, and irregular microvascular structure. The final diagnosis was a well-differentiated adenocarcinoma that remained in the mucosa and was not accompanied by dysplasia

the lesion (2.6) were extracted as significant findings suggestive of neoplastic lesions. These results suggest that it is important to focus on superficial lesions without ulceration in endoscopic diagnosis of UCAN, and that regular microsurface structures and irregular microvascular structures under image-enhanced observation may be useful in diagnosing neoplastic lesions. However, the agreement of the findings among observers was only moderate, and the reproducibility of the above findings has not been confirmed.

Thus, efforts for endoscopic diagnosis of UCAN are being made worldwide. However, the endoscopic findings of UCAN are much more diverse than those of ordinary colorectal cancer, and the relationship between these findings and histopathological images has not been sufficiently investigated. On the other hand, a project on UCAN endoscopic diagnosis using more detailed magnified endoscopic findings than FACILE and endoscopic treatment strategies is underway in Japan, and various magnified endoscopic findings characteristic of UC have been proposed. We believe that the characteristics of inflammatory bowel disease-associated cancers described in this book will provide important information not only for clinical practice but also for research in this field in the future.

5 Conclusion

We have described the current status and future development of endoscopic diagnosis of UCAN by introducing two projects, SCENIC and FACILE. We hope that you will understand the characteristics of UCAN by carefully reading the cases in this book along with this information.

References

1. Riddell RH, Goldman H, Ransohoff DF, et al. Dysplasia in inflammatory bowel disease: standardized classification with provisional clinical applications. Hum Pathol. 1983;14:931–68.
2. Beaugerie L, Itzkowitz SH. Cancers complicating inflammatory bowel disease. N Engl J Med. 2015;372:1441–52.
3. Laine L, Kaltenbach T, Barkun A, et al. SCENIC international consensus statement on surveillance and management of dysplasia in inflammatory bowel disease. Gastrointest Endosc. 2015;81:489–501.
4. Laine L, Kaltenbach T, Barkun A, et al. SCENIC international consensus statement on surveillance and management of dysplasia in inflammatory bowel disease. Gastroenterology. 2015;148:639–51.
5. Workshop PitP. The Paris endoscopic classification of superficial neoplastic lesions: esophagus, stomach, and colon. Gastrointest Endosc. 2003;58:S3–43.
6. Feueustein JD, Rakowsky S, Sattler L, et al. Meta-analysis of dye-based chromoendoscopy compared with standard- and high-definition white light endoscopy in patients with inflammatory bowel disease at increased risk of colon cancer. Gastrointest Endosc. 2019;90:186–95.
7. Bisschops R, Bessissow T, Dekker E, et al. Pit pattern analysis with high-definition chromoendoscopy and narrow-band imaging for optical diagnosis of dysplasia in patients with ulcerative colitis. Gastrointest Endosc. 2017;86:1100–6.
8. Mohan BP, Khan SR, Chandan S, et al. Endoscopic resection of colon dysplasia in patients with inflammatory bowel disease: a systematic review and meta-analysis. Gastrointest Endosc. 2021;93:59–67.
9. Watanabe T, Ajioka Y, Mitsuyama K, et al. Comparison of targeted vs random biopsies for surveillance of ulcerative colitis-associated colorectal. Gastroenterology. 2016;151:1122–30.
10. Moussata D, Allez M, Cazals-Hatem D, et al. Are random biopsies still useful for the detection of neoplasia in patients with IBD undergoing surveillance colonoscopy with chromoendoscopy? Gut. 2017;67:616–24.
11. Chiu K, Riddell RH, Schaeffer DF. DALM, rest in peace: a pathologist's perspective on dysplasia in inflammatory bowel disease in the post-DALM era. Mod Pathol. 2018;31:1180–90.
12. Iacucci M, McQuaid K, Gui XS, et al. Multimodal (FACILE) classification for optical diagnosis of inflammatory bowel disease associated neoplasia. Endoscopy. 2019;51:133–41.

Crohn's Disease-Associated Lower Gastrointestinal Cancer

Kitaro Futami

1 Introduction

Crohn's disease (CD) carries the same risk of carcinogenesis as ulcerative colitis (UC) [1], and the number of CD-associated cancer cases is increasing in Japan concurrent with an increase in the number of long-term cases [2]. However, the number of CD cases complicated with cancer is much lower than that of UC cases complicated with cancer. Additionally, the morphological analysis of CD-associated gastrointestinal cancers is not as advanced because the entire gastrointestinal tract is at risk; endoscopy is limited by stenosis, fistulae, and anal lesions; and frequency of CD-associated cancers is high in the rectal and anal regions, where gastroenterologists are least familiar. In this chapter, we present our experience with CD-associated lower gastrointestinal cancers and describe current issues, focusing on diagnosis [3]. The description of the presented cases is included in Sect. 3 of the text, and the corresponding cases are indicated by (). The description of cancer lesions is based on the 9th edition of the Japanese Classification of Colorectal, Appendiceal, and Anal Carcinoma [4].

2 Examination of Cases in Our Institution

Up to December 2020, 45 (6.3%) of the 711 CD patients treated surgically for bowel lesions at our institution had lower gastrointestinal malignancies: seven cases of small intestine cancer, four of colon cancer, 29 of rectal and anal cancer, and six of rectal carcinoid tumor (one of these patients also had ascending colon cancer), all of which were small lesions (<10 mm). Three tumors were endoscopically resected and three were diagnosed based on findings of pathological examinations after intestinal resection. The following studies were performed for all tumors except carcinoid tumors.

K. Futami (✉)
Center for Clinical Medical Research (Surgery), Fukuoka University Chikushi Hospital, Chikushino, Japan

2.1 Comparison with Conventional Sporadic Lower Gastrointestinal Cancer (Table 1)

A total of 2333 non-CD lower gastrointestinal sporadic cancers treated in our department up to December 2014 were compared with CD-associated cancers. The risk of small intestine cancer was much higher in CD cases [5], as was the risk of rectal and anal cancer. There was a large difference in the distribution of primary cancer sites between CD-associated cancers and sporadic lower gastrointestinal cancers. Patients with CD-associated cancers were more than 10 years younger at the time of cancer diagnosis than patients with sporadic cancers.

Table 1 Crohn's disease associated lower gastrointestinal cancers compared with sporadic cancers

	Crohn's disease-associated cancer [40 cases]	Sporadic cancer [2333 cases]
Tumor site		
Small intestine cancer	17.5% [7]	0.4% [10]
Colon cancer	10.0% [4]	57.2% [1335]
Rectal and anal cancer	72.5% [29]	42.3% [988]
Age at diagnosis (years)		
Small intestine cancer	46.0	58.6
Colon cancer	50.0	67.7
Rectal and anal cancer	48.7	64.8
Gross type (Type 3, 4, 5)	62.5% [25]	8.7% [203]
Histological type (poorly differentiated)	65.0% [26]	14.5% [339]
Curative resection (R0)	65.0% [26]	82.4% [1922]

T. Matsui et al. (eds.), *Atlas of Inflammatory Bowel Disease-Associated Intestinal Cancer*,
https://doi.org/10.1007/978-981-19-3413-1_3

We also compared gross morphology and histopathological findings of the tumors. CD patients tended to have more invasive tumor types (types 3, 4, and 5) and poorly differentiated histologies (poorly differentiated adenocarcinoma, mucinous carcinoma, and signet ring cell carcinoma). Additionally, the curative resection rate was low, reflecting the high malignant potential of cancer [6].

2.2 Clinical Aspects of CD-Associated Lower Gastrointestinal Tract Cancer (Table 2)

Clinical factors, including tumor site, age, sex, basic CD type, symptoms, and timing of medical examination, of 40 cases of lower gastrointestinal cancer in CD patients were compared. The frequencies are calculated based on the entire cohort of 711 CD patients who underwent surgery. CD-associated cancers were more common in women, and patients with CD in both the small and large intestines were more likely to develop tumors. Among patients with small intestine CD, three cases of anal canal cancer were observed. The averagess duration of CD among patients who developed cancer was more than 20 years, and 32 of 40 patients had a history of intestinal surgery. Regarding the timing of cancer diagnosis, there was only one case of preoperative diagnosis of small intestine cancer; however, three cases of colon cancer and 24 of 27 resected cases of rectal and anal cancer were diagnosed preoperatively.

3 CD-Associated Small Intestine Cancer

3.1 Analysis of Cases in Our Institution (Table 3)

All patients had ileal cancer, including one patient (small and large intestine (SL) type) who underwent surgery at another institution. One of the six patients treated at our department was a 40-year-old man who was referred for treatment of refractory multiple anal fistulas, which were successfully treated with seton's drainage and biologic agents; however, he subsequently developed anal stenosis. Seven years after cancer surveillance every year, an erythematous polyp was found in the oral side of the anastomosis after ileocecal resection of ileal stenosis, and atypical epithelium was detected by biopsy (Case 1). Ileal cancer complicated with overt ileus in two patients was diagnosed intraoperatively and resected without complete cure owing to peritoneal dissemination. One patient had high tumor marker levels, and PET/computed tomography showed fluorodeoxyglucose accumulation; however, it was difficult to distinguish the tumor from inflammation, and an endoscope could not reach the ileal lesion. The other patient had severe ileus, and contrast radiography using the ileus tube and CT could not distinguish it from a CD lesion (Case 2). The patient had two cancerous lesions, one at the stenosis and the other at the blind loop after bypass surgery, which is considered a risk factor for cancer complications [7].

Table 2 Crohn's disease-associated lower gastrointestinal cancer: clinical features in 40 cases

		Small intestine cancer [7]	Colon cancer [4]	Rectal and anal cancer [29]
Frequency (vs. 711 surgical cases)		1.0%	0.6%	4.1%
Age at diagnosis of cancer (years)		46.0	50.0	48.7
Sex	Male (502)	0.8% (4)	0.6% (3)	3.2% (16)
	Female (209)	1.4% (3)	0.5% (1)	6.2% (13)
Type of CD	Small intestine type (268 cases)	0.4% (1)	0%	1.1% (3)
	Small and large intestine type (391)	1.5% (6)	0.8% (3)	6.1% (24)
	Large intestine type (52)	0% (0)	1.9% (1)	3.8% (2)
Duration of CD (months)		235	226	293
Previous bowel surgery		6 (85.7%)	1 (25.0%)	25 (86.2%)
Timing of medical examination	Preoperative	1	3	24
	During surgery	2	1	0
	Postoperative	3	0	3
	Non-surgical	1 (palpated cervical LN)	0	2 (liver metastasis and dissemination)

Table 3 Crohn's disease-associated small intestine cancer: clinical and pathological features in 7 cases

Multiplicity of the ileal lesion	Single: 5, multiple: 2 (1 patient with 2 lesions and 1 patients with 4 lesions)
Pathological findings	Ia Tis well-differentiated (with atypical epithelium) by surveillance diagnosis
	IIb Tis well-differentiated IIc T1a well-differentiated+ IIa Tis well-differentiated 3 lesions [with atypical epithelium]
	Type 1 T2 well-differentiated Type 3, T4a, well- to moderately differentiated, 2 lesions P(+) Type 4 T3 well-differentiated P(+) Type 3 Tx well- and poorly differentiated M(LN) (nonresectable)
Cancer symptoms	Ileus symptoms 4, no symptoms 3
Crohn's disease	Stenotic lesion 9, non-stenotic lesion 1, intestinal lesion at blind loop after bypass 1
Small intestine endoscopy	Biopsy diagnosis 2, unable to biopsy 1
Small bowel radiography	Suspected cancer 1, definite Crohn's lesion 5
Imaging examination	Cancer diagnosis CT 0/6, MRI 0/1, PET 1/1 (cancer suspicion)
Tumor markers	Positive CEA 1/5, positive CA1-9 2/5

In two patients, early-stage cancer was diagnosed in the periphery of longitudinal ulcers of the stenosis based on postoperative pathological findings. One patient had four lesions, but they were small lesions that could not be diagnosed as carcinomas even based on pathological examinations of the resected specimen (Case 3). In one patient who did not undergo surgery, primary ileal cancer was confirmed by small bowel endoscopy after metastasis to the left cervical lymph node (Case 5). The morphology of the three early-stage cancers included one stage IIc submucosally invasive (SM) carcinoma and five elevated mucosal carcinomas. All lesions were well-differentiated adenocarcinomas, and two lesions had concomitant atypical epithelium in the surrounding mucosa. In addition, all seven carcinomas were located within severely stenotic lesions.

3.2 Diagnosis of CD-Associated Small Intestine Cancer

Although the frequency of CD-associated small intestine cancer is low, the relative risk of small intestine cancer is very high in CD patients, and it is predominantly found in the ileum [5]. It is often very difficult to diagnose preoperatively [8, 9]. We used several different methods to diagnose CD-associated small intestine cancer in our patients. Tumor marker (CEA, CA19-9) levels were examined preoperatively in five patients, two of whom were diagnosed with stage IV disease. Therefore, tumor marker assessment may be useful for cancer detection, but it cannot identify early-stage disease [10]. Imaging can also be used for diagnosis. PET showed accumulation in the lesion in only one patient, but a small bowel endoscope could not reach the lesion owing to stenosis and adhesions. CT and MRI did not lead to a diagnosis of cancer owing to the severely stenotic lesion. Therefore, other imaging studies may be needed in these patients. However, double-balloon small bowel endoscopy is not suitable for surveillance because of its invasiveness and difficulty in reaching the lesion, and capsule endoscopy is not suitable for stenotic lesions and cannot be performed. In the future, biopsy of abnormal findings should be performed during endoscopy (as in Case 4), and a diagnostic method that combines contrast-enhanced ultrasonography [11] with CT, MRI, and PET is needed [12]. In particular, in patients with a long disease course, systematic imaging studies should always be performed considering the possibility of cancer, and in refractory cases, surgery should be considered as a preventive measure.

The principle of surgical treatment for CD is minimal resection or strictureplasty to eliminate complications and preserve the bowel. Conversely, for cancer, wide resection, including lymph node dissection, is standard. Therefore, the techniques are conflicting. Given these conflicting priorities, intraoperative diagnosis should be the goal, along with rapid pathological diagnosis of cancer is suspected [13]. The most problematic issue is the treatment of patients who are diagnosed postoperatively. In this series, two patients were diagnosed postoperatively, and although no additional surgery was performed because they had early-stage cancer, reoperation was considered if the cancer was advanced. The presence or absence of lymph node metastasis is a factor for determining the suitability of additional surgery, and routine pathological examination of the lymph nodes, which is also useful for detecting non-caseating epithelioid granuloma, is a recommended measure [3].

4 CD-Associated Colorectal and Anal Cancer

4.1 Analysis of Cases in Our Institution (Tables 4 and 5)

There were four CD patients with colon cancer in our institution: three men and one woman, among whom three were undergoing surgery for the first time. One case of ascending colon cancer was diagnosed by endoscopy based on symptoms of abdominal pain and bleeding (type 2, well to moderately differentiated adenocarcinoma, III A: P0H0N1SE), and one case was diagnosed by endoscopy because of a chief complaint of abdominal pain after 3 years without a regular visit (Case 7). In a patient with a transverse colon lesion with ileus, cancer was strongly suspected based on scirrhous-like contrast radiography findings; however, the diagnosis could not be made by biopsy because of severe stenosis and covering by noncancerous tissue. The diagnosis was confirmed intraoperatively (Case 8). A sigmoid colon tumor was diagnosed by preoperative colonoscopy of recurrent ileal CD lesions, and it was SM cancer with no cancer-related symptoms (Case 6). In all four patients, no atypical epithelium was found in the surrounding mucosa on pathological examination of serial sections. All patients underwent curative resection; however, two patients with advanced cancer relapsed owing to peritoneal dissemination.

We had 29 patients with CD who developed rectal and anal cancer [14, 15]. In this series, rectal and anal cancers were more common in women. The disease type of CD was as follows: three small intestine type, 24 small and large intestine type, and two large intestine type. Twenty patients had previously undergone intestinal surgery (range, 1–4) and 27 had anal lesions. The tumor location was the upper rectum in three cases, and 24 tumors, including those in the lower rectum, had invaded the anal canal. Twenty-four patients were preoperatively diagnosed. Twenty-seven patients underwent surgical treatment; one patient of two had Rb (type 3, poorly differentiated adenocarcinoma) which was diagnosed as multiple liver metastases and the other had

Table 4 Crohn's disease-associated colon cancer: clinical and pathological features in 4 cases

Lesion site	Ascending colon 2, transverse colon 1, sigmoid colon 1
Pathological findings	Ascending colon [IIIa] type 2 T4a well differentiated Ascending colon [IIIc] type 3 T4a mucinous Transverse colon [IIIc] type 3 T4a mucinous Sigmoid colon [I] Is T1a well differentiated
Cancer symptoms	Ascending colon: 1 patient with abdominal pain + anemia and 1 patient with abdominal pain + increased frequency of defecation
	Transverse colon 1 with ileus
	Sigmoid colon 1 without symptom
Endoscopic biopsy	Cancer diagnosis 3/4 [1 unable to diagnose as cancer]
Contrast-enhanced enterography	Cancerous lesion 4/4
Imaging tests	Cancer diagnosis using CT 1/4, using MRI 1/1
Tumor markers	Positive CEA 0/4, positive CA19–9 0/4

Table 5 Crohn's disease-associated rectal and anal cancer: clinical and pathological features in 29 cases

Occupied area	Ra 3, Rb 2, RbP 9, PRb 6, P 9		
Gross type	Type 0: 4, Type 1: 2, Type 2: 2, Type 3: 3, Type 4: 6, Type 5: 11, Unknown: 1		
Pathological findings	Well-differentiated 6, well- to moderately differentiated 1, well- to poorly differentiated (mucinous) 2		
	Moderately to poorly differentiated 2, Poorly differentiated (mucinous) 1, signet ring cell 1		
	Mucinous 15, Poorly differentiated neuroendocrine 1		
Stage	0: 4, I: 0, IIa: 10, IIb: 1, IIc: 2, IIIa:, 0, IIIb: 1, IIIc: 4, IV: 7		
With cancer symptoms	20 cases (pain 15, bleeding 4, mucus discharge 4, etc.)		
Diagnosis	Transanal biopsy 13, endoscopic biopsy 12, postoperative 3, cytology 1		
Imaging findings	Carcinoma lesion	Cancer or inflammation	No lesion
CT	9/26 (34.6%)	4/26 (15.4%)	13/26 (50.0%)
MRI	6/19 (31.6%)	6/19 (31.6%)	8/19 (42.1%)
PET	1/3 (33.3%)	2/3 (66.7%)	0/3 (0%)
Positive tumor markers	CEA 14/29 (48.3%); CA-19-9 5/27 (18.5%)		
Surgical treatment	Resection 24 (R0 18; R1, 5; R2, 1), non-resection 5		

a nonoperative case of peritoneal dissemination (type 4, mucinous carcinoma). There were four cases of mucosal carcinoma: two cases of IIa, one case of IIb, and one case of Isp + IIb [case 18], all of which were flat to elevated well-differentiated adenocarcinomas. Three cases were complicated with atypical epithelium in the surrounding mucosa. Of the 25 advanced cancers, 20 were invasive (types 3, 4, and 5), and 16 of the 21 poorly differentiated cancers had a mucinous component. In terms of cancer stage, 12 cases were stage IIIa or higher with lymph node metastasis, and of the 24 resections (resection rate 82.8%), 18 were curative resections (R0) (curative resection rate 62.1%). There were many cases of local invasion, and 10 of 24 resections required combined resection of adjacent organs (Cases 10 and19). Three of the five unresected cases were highly locally invasive with distant metastasis.

4.2 Comparison of Rectal and Anal Cancers with and without Cancer-Related Symptoms (Table 6)

Among 29 patients with rectal and anal cancer, 20 were diagnosed because of cancer-related symptoms. Symptoms included persistent pain in 15 patients, mucus discharge in four patients, and bleeding in four patients; the average duration from symptom onset to diagnosis was 4.2 months. Sclerosis and tenderness were prominent on palpation. All patients had advanced cancer, and 12 patients had stage IIIa or more lymph node positivity. In one patient, rectal wash cytology was performed, and the diagnosis was stage IIIa cancer (Case 13). Thirteen patients had elevated tumor marker levels. In 10 patients, imaging studies (CT and MRI) indicated cancerous lesions, but in four patients, the tumor could not be differentiated from CD lesions. In one patient diagnosed after colorectal anastomosis, additional resection was needed. Preoperative endoscopy was negative in multiple biopsies, but pathological examination of the resected rectum after rectal amputation showed early-stage cancer.

Among the nine patients without cancer symptoms, six had cancer that was diagnosed endoscopically, and the lesions included two cases of villous mucosa (Cases 12 and 14), one case of erythematous irregular mucosa (Case 9), one case of erythematous polyp (Case 18), one case of mild elevated lesion, and one case of flat erythema. Two cases of anorectal dysfunction owing to multiple anorectal surgeries were diagnosed based on histological findings after amputation. None of the patients had lymph node metastasis, and one patient with intramucosal well-differentiated adenocarcinoma of the anal canal had high CEA levels that normalized after surgery.

Five of 20 patients with cancer symptoms had unresectable tumors, and resection of adjacent organs was required in 10 of the remaining 15 patients, including six patients in whom total pelvic organ resection was performed. Nine patients underwent R0 resection, five underwent R1 resection, and one underwent R2 resection; 10 of the 15 patients developed postoperative recurrence. None of the nine patients without cancer symptoms required resection of adjacent organs. Among these nine patients, the mean observation period was 107.3 months (16–337 months), and only one patient (stage IIa) developed local recurrence at 35 months postoperatively [16].

The ECCO guidelines state that anal canal carcinoma is frequently associated with anal fistula [17]. Therefore, it is often incorrectly assumed that anal canal carcinoma originates from an anal fistula. However, we only observed fistula tract origin based on pathological findings of one patient (Case 17). The diagnosis of mucinous carcinoma was made from the excised tissue of the fistula tract, and the lesion was small, making diagnosis difficult without the help of an experienced pathologist. Serial sections of the resected specimen showed that the mucosa of the anal canal was associated with a very well-differentiated adenocarci-

Table 6 Crohn's disease-associated rectal and anal cancer in 29 cases: comparison of cases with and without symptoms

	Cancer with symptoms (20 cases)	Cancer without symptoms (9 cases)
Ra/Rb/RbP/PRb/P	2/1/7/6/4	1/1/2/0/5
Stage : 0 + I/IIa + b + IIc/IIIa + IIIb + IIIc/IV	0/8/5/7	4/5/0/0
Biopsy diagnosis:		
endoscopy	6	6
transanal	13 (cytology 1)	1
postoperative	1	2
Duration of cancer symptoms (months)	4.2 (1–21)	
Imaging findings (cancerous lesion)	CT 9/19 • MRI6/15 • PET 1/1	CT 0/7 • MRI 0/4 • PET 0/2
Positive tumor markers	13/20	1/9
Surgical treatment	Resection 15 (R0 9), nonresection 5	Reaction9 (R0 9)
combined resection of adjacent organs	10	0
combined resection of CD lesion	5	1

noma, which provides valuable insight into the carcinogenic matrix of CD-associated anal canal cancer. In addition, there was no atypical epithelium in the fistulous tracts of a patient with early-stage carcinoma (Case 18). Carcinoma of the anal ulcer (Case 16) and two mass-type carcinomas were derived from the rectal mucosa and not from the fistulous tract.

4.3 Diagnosis of Colorectal and Anal Cancer

Endoscopic surveillance is recommended for CD-associated colorectal cancer same as UC [18]. However, stenosis, fistulae, and intractable anal lesions owing to CD lesions are obstacles to endoscopic examination of the final decision. Fortunately, three of the patients with colon cancer in our study were undergoing surgery for the first time and had mild anorectal lesions. All patients were diagnosed by endoscopic biopsy in a regular outpatient clinic.

In typical cases, the rectal-anal region is directly palpable and cancer can be suspected based on gross findings in the anal region (Case 10). Even if there are no findings around the anus, tenderness and sclerosis by palpation during digital rectal examination are also considered important findings of cancer (Cases 11 and 20).

Cancer of the rectum and anal canal is common in Japan, and cancer surveillance by transanal and endoscopic biopsy has been investigated. Endoscopic findings include inflamed mucosa [19], erythematous polyps, and erythematous lesions. If there are suspicious findings, as in Case 9, the biopsy site should be carefully considered and biopsy should be repeated. To detect cancer at an early stage by endoscopy, lesions should be targeted for biopsy, as discussed for UC cases.

Based on our experience, it is essential to diagnose tumors before they progress past stage II and metastasize to the lymph nodes in order to prevent excessive surgical burden and lead to good prognosis. Although some reports [6] have identified changes in symptoms, such as pain and mucous stools, as triggers for cancer diagnosis, cancer is already quite advanced when symptoms appear, and the diagnosis of cancer at a stage without cancer symptoms is a prerequisite for improving patient prognosis [16]. We previously reported the usefulness of biopsy of the anorectal region [10]. However, targeted biopsy by endoscopy is the most important tool for the diagnosis of early-stage cancer, and close cooperation among internal medicine specialists, surgeons, proctologists, and pathologists is essential for early diagnosis, such as for simultaneous anal dilatation and endoscopy under anesthesia for cases of anal stenosis that are difficult to examine in an outpatient setting.

5 Conclusion

Cancer is an infrequent complication of CD, but it is an important complication with a direct impact on life expectancy. The prognosis of CD patients with cancer is worse than that of patients with conventional sporadic cancers, and the onset of cancer at a young age is deeply related to quality of life; therefore, the establishment of a surveillance method combining various examinations with the analysis of lesions is urgently needed. In addition to identifying a multidisciplinary treatment method in collaboration with medical oncologists and radiologists, it will be necessary to study indications for surgery for refractory lesions to prevent cancer.

Finally, we hope that this book will lead to progress in the treatment of CD-associated cancers.

References

1. Zisman TL, Rubin DT. Colorectal cancer and dysplasia in inflammatory bowel disease. World J Gastroenterol. 2008;14:2662–9.
2. Higashi D, Katsuno H, Kimura H, et al. Current state of and problems related to cancer of the intestinal tract associated with Crohn's disease in Japan. Anticancer Res. 2016;36(7):3761–6.
3. Futami K, Higashi D, Hirano Y, et al. Surgery for cancer complicated by Crohn's disease. Surgery. 2017;71:1029–38. (in Japanese)
4. Sugihara K, editor. Japanese classification of colorectal, appendiceal, anal carcinoma. 9th ed. Tokyo: Kanehara Shuppan; 2018.
5. Canavan C, Abrams KR, Mayberry J. Meta-analysis: colorectal and small bowel cancer risk in patients with Crohn's disease. Aliment Pharmacol Ther. 2006;23:1097–104.
6. Sugita A, Koganei K, Tatsumi K, et al. Rectal and anal canal carcinoma associated with Crohn's disease. J Jpn Soc Gastroenterol. 2013;110(3):396–402. (in Japanese)
7. Greenstein AJ, Sachar D, Pucillo A, et al. Cancer in Crohn's disease after diversionary surgery. A report of seven carcinomas occurring in the excluded bowel. Am J Surg. 1978;135:86–90.
8. Piton G, Cosnes J, Monnet E, et al. Risk factors associated with small bowel adenocarcinoma in Crohn's disease: a case-control study. Am J Gastroenterol. 2008;103(7):1730–6.
9. Ikeuchi H, Uchino M, Matsuoka H, et al. Cancer of Crohn's disease and future measures. Intestine. 2010;14:505–10. (in Japanese)
10. Futami K, Higashi J, Egawa Y, et al. Diagnosis, treatment, and prognosis of patients with carcinoma of Crohn's disease. Gastroenterol Surg. 2013;36(1):97–105. (in Japanese)
11. Hata J, Imamura Y, Manabe N, et al. Extracorporeal ultrasound of the gastrointestinal tract. Stomach Intestine. 2016;51(7):917–26. (in Japanese)
12. Noguchi A, Watanabe N, Ajioka Y, et al. A case of Crohn's disease-related small bowel cancer with recurrence. Stomach Intestine. 2014;49(9):1339–45. (in Japanese)
13. Sugita A, Koganei K, Tatsumi K, et al. Surgical treatment of small bowel cancer complicated by Crohn's disease. Intestine. 2015;19(4):399–404. (in Japanese)
14. Thomas M, Bienkowski R, Vandermeer TJ, et al. Malignant transformation in perianal fistulas of Crohn's disease: a systematic review of the literature. J Gastrointest Surg. 2010;14:66–73.
15. Yano Y, Matsui T, Uno H, et al. Risks and clinical features of colorectal cancer complicating Crohn's disease in Japanese patients. J Gastroenterol Hepatol. 2008;23:1683–8.

16. Hirano Y, Futami K, Higashi D, et al. Anorectal cancer surveillance in Crohn's disease. J Anus Rectum Colon. 2018;2(4):145–54.
17. Annese V, Beaugeric L, Egan L, et al. European evidence-based consensus: inflammatory bowel disease and malignancies. J Crohns Colitis. 2015;9(11):945–65.
18. Freidman S, Rubin PH, Bodian C, et al. Screening and surveillance colonoscopy in chronic Crohn's colitis: results of a surveillance program spanning 25years. Clin Gastroenterol Hepatol. 2008;6:993–8.
19. Esaki M, Ikegami K, Kawachi S, et al. Characteristics of malignant diseases of the gastrointestinal tract; malignant diseases of the small intestine and colon. Stomach Intestine. 2012;47(10):1545–57. (In Japanese)

Clinicopathological Features and Pathological Diagnosis of Inflammatory Bowel Disease-Associated Cancer

Akinori Iwashita and Hiroshi Tanabe

1 Introduction

Ulcerative colitis (UC)-associated carcinoma and Crohn's disease (CD)-associated carcinoma have distinct clinicopathological features. Concerning the site of carcinoma, UC-associated carcinoma has mainly occurred in the rectosigmoid area of total colitis type, and UC-associated carcinoma has a tendency to occur in multiple cancers of the colon. On the other hand, CD-associated cancers in Japan are predominantly solitary mucinous carcinomas occurring in the rectum and anus. The histological features of both types of carcinoma are similar and have variety, ranging from very well-differentiated adenocarcinoma to poorly differentiated adenocarcinoma with a background of dysplasia. Reflecting the variety of histology and the high degree of inflammation in the background, the gross image also shows a variety of complex morphologies, and the boundaries between them are unclear. In the following, we will review the morphological characteristics and pathological diagnosis of inflammatory bowel disease (IBD)-associated cancers with case examples.

2 Gross Characteristics of Inflammatory Bowel Disease (IBD)-Associated Cancer

Common gross features of IBD-associated cancers include (1) difficulty in recognizing the lesion, (2) atypical gross appearance, and (3) difficulty in diagnosing the extent and depth of the lesion. In other words, it is not a single shape like ordinary sporadic carcinoma, but a complex variety with indistinct borders. This may be due to both background factors, such as inflammation, ulceration and scarring, fistulas, and inflammatory polyps, as well as the nature of the tumor itself, including the presence of dysplasia, tumor differentiation, presentation, mode of invasion, and extracellular mucous degeneration. At our institution, all specimens from patients with IBD are divided in a staircase pattern, and in patients with cancer, all sections are carefully examined. Therefore, some early-stage cancers are detected only after postoperative histopathological examination.

UC-related cancers are often widespread, including dysplasia, whereas most CD-associated cancers are confined to a relatively small area. This may be attributed to the difference between the continuous and diffuse inflammation of UC and the discontinuous and disproportionate inflammation of CD.

2.1 Gross Features of Ulcerative Colitis (UC)-Associated Cancer

Most early-stage cancers are raised, flat, or a mixture of the two (UC cases 2–7). Basically, due to the presence of background inflammation and dysplasia, the boundary with the surrounding non-tumor mucosa is extremely obscure, making it difficult to diagnose the extent of the lesion or even its presence, and some lesions are quite extensive (UC cases 5, 6). Most sporadic advanced colorectal cancers are of the ulcerative-expansive type (type 2), whereas ulcerative-infiltrative type (type 3) and diffuse-infiltrative type (type 4) are more common in UC-associated advanced cancers. At our institution, unclassified type (type 5) and apparently early-stage cancer-like lesions are common. Sporadic carcinoma usually shows expansive growth (massive invasion, potato-like invasion), and ischemic necrosis, prolapse, and ulceration of the lesion due to damage to the vascular

A. Iwashita (✉)
Fukuoka University, Fukuoka, Japan
e-mail: iwa-aki@fukuoka-u.ac.jp

H. Tanabe
Department of Pathology, Fukuoka University Chikushi Hospital, Chikushino, Japan

T. Matsui et al. (eds.), *Atlas of Inflammatory Bowel Disease-Associated Intestinal Cancer*,
https://doi.org/10.1007/978-981-19-3413-1_4

network. However, in many cases of UC-associated cancers, the original layered structure of the intestinal wall is maintained because the intramucosal lesions remain without ulceration and grow diffusely (scattered infiltration, root-like infiltration) in the deep part of the intestinal wall (UC cases 12, 15). There are also lesions that appear to be early-stage cancers even in advanced cancers because of deep extracellular mucous degeneration and lack of fibrous stromal reaction (UC case 10). These growth and invasion patterns are thought to be involved in the formation of a variety of gross forms.

2.2 Gross Features of Crohn's Disease (CD)-Associated Cancer

CD-associated colorectal cancers are overwhelmingly advanced cancers originating in the rectum and anus, most of which are mucinous carcinomas (CD cases 10–12, 15, 17, 19, 20). Some cases are presumed to have arisen from perianal fistulas (CD cases 17, 19). In many cases, the anal region is high degree stenosis, making the diagnosis of cancer clinically difficult. In addition, some very well-differentiated adenocarcinomas are difficult to diagnose by biopsy, and frequent biopsies are necessary to confirm the diagnosis. At our institution, most of the CD-associated cancers in the rectum and anus are type 5. In other portions, there are lesions with type 3 (CD cases 7, 8) and lesions with type 5 due to the effect of inherent inflammatory changes of CD such as background non-neoplastic inflammatory polyps and ulcer scars (CD case 9), but in any case, mucinous carcinomas are histologically as common as lesions in the recto-anal region.

In Japan, small bowel cancer is not a common complication, but its gross type is mostly type 3 or 4 advanced cancer, which is difficult to distinguish from inflammatory changes or stenosis of CD (CD case 5), and cancer may be pathologically diagnosed by rapid intraoperative diagnosis (CD case 2). Early-stage carcinoma of the small intestine is modified by inflammation and ulceration of the CD and is very difficult to detect preoperatively (CD case 3), and even when it presents as an elevated lesion, it is not easy to distinguish from inflammatory polyps (CD case 1).

3 Histopathological Characteristics of Inflammatory Bowel Disease (IBD) (UC, CD)-Associated Cancers

Histopathological features of IBD-associated cancers include (1) a high incidence of lesions with dysplasia, (2) a variety of histological features including very well- and poorly differentiated adenocarcinomas and a mixture of both, (3) a high incidence of mucinous carcinoma or partial extracellular mucous degeneration, and (4) a high incidence of lesions with immunohistochemically gastric mucin phenotype. These features are common to both UC-associated and CD-associated cancers.

Originally, the concept of dysplasia of the gastrointestinal tract in Europe and the United States included epithelial tumors without invasion, i.e., adenomas and carcinomas, unlike in Japan. Based on this basic concept, in 1983, the Inflammatory Bowel Disease-Dysplasia Study Group (IBD-DMSG) of Riddell et al. [1] defined dysplasia in patients with UC as an obvious neoplastic change in the colonic epithelium and stated that it could be considered a marker of precancerous lesions or a cancer risk factor in UC. They recommended the classification of dysplasia, which is now widely used in the United States and Europe. By the way, dysplasia can be seen not only in UC but also in CD.

On the other hand, in Japan, the histopathological classification of atypical epithelium occurring in the mucosa of UC by the Research Group on Intractable Inflammatory Bowel Disease of Specified Diseases of the Ministry of Health and Welfare [2] is often used. This classification distinguishes lesions that can be diagnosed as intramucosal carcinoma from dysplasia. However, in practice, it is often difficult to differentiate between regenerative atypical epithelium and dysplasia, and between dysplasia and noninvasive intramucosal carcinoma, and there is no clear boundary between dysplasia and noninvasive intramucosal carcinoma. This differentiation is quite problematic for pathologists because there are a lot of diagnostic disagreements between pathologists in Japan and also in West. In particular, it is extremely difficult to make these determinations based on biopsy materials alone. In the present study, the cases at our institution were classified as dysplastic epithelium, which corresponds to UC-IIb (more suspicious for neoplastic changes) and UC-III (neoplastic changes but cannot be judged as cancer) of the histopathological classification of atypical epithelium in UC of the abovementioned Ministry of Health and Welfare group study, excluding obvious adenomas. In cases where the borderline diagnosis between intramucosal carcinoma and dysplasia was difficult, both were mapped together (UC cases 6, 10, 16).

Differentiated carcinomas seen in IBD-associated cancers are very well-differentiated adenocarcinomas, meaning that atypia is very weak, and many lesions show cellular differentiation, such as goblet cells, endocrine cells, and Paneth cells. Therefore, a definite diagnosis of atypia (cancer, inflammation, or dysplasia) is sometimes quite difficult when biopsied material is obtained from the superficial part of the mucosa. We often experienced cases in which a definite diagnosis was possible when tumor invasion to the submucosal layer was observed after postoperative examination (Fig. 11d, e in the Case 14 of Chap. 7). Although poorly differentiated adenocarcinoma and signet ring cell carcinoma are also frequent in CD-associated cancers, IBD-associated cancers often present with mixed histology of poorly to very well-differentiated adenocarcinoma rather than single histology. (UC cases 1, 2, 17, CD cases 7, 9, 15, 20). There are frequently mucinous carcinoma components including extracellular mucous degeneration in IBD-associated carcinoma. We can suppose that there may be similarities in the pathogenesis of IBD-associated carcinomas and common sporadic mucinous carcinomas.

Ajioka et al. [3] found that MUC5AC was expressed in the cancerous area and surrounding nontumor mucosa of patients with long-term and total colitis type UC, suggesting that gastric metaplasia of the colonic mucosa occurs due to chronic persistent inflammation at the preliminary stage of carcinogenesis. In our case series [4], 63.5% of UC-associated cancers were MUC5AC-positive, i.e., they showed a mixed gastric and intestinal mucin phenotype, which was higher than that of 20% of normal sporadic rectal cancers. Therefore, the presence of mixed gastric mucin phenotype may be useful in differentiating IBD-related cancer from sporadic cancer (UC cases 2–4, 10, CD cases 6, 18).

4 Conclusion

The clinicopathological characteristics and pathological diagnosis of IBD-associated cancers are reviewed with case examples. IBD- associated cancers are characterized by borderline indistinctness, a great variety of gross and histological images, and immunohistochemical evidence of mixed gastric and intestinal mucin phenotype. Therefore, it is advisable to divide the all resected specimen into staircase-like sections and examine all the sections carefully. However, even with the experience of many cases, the diagnosis is still not easy and profound. In particular, biopsy diagnosis should be performed carefully and appropriately with the utmost care and in close consultation with the clinician.

References

1. Riddell RH, Goldman H, Ransohoff DF, et al. Dysplasia in inflammatory bowel disease: standardized classification with provisional clinical applications. Hum Pathol. 1983;14:931–68.
2. Mutoh T, Wakasa H, Kina I, et al. Pathological criteria for atypical epithelium appearing in ulcerative colitis - proposal of new criteria for application to surveillance colonoscopy. J Jpn Soc Coloproctol. 1994;47:547–51. (in Japanese)
3. Ajioka Y, Iwanaga A, Watanabe J, et al. Histogenesis of colorectal cancer in ulcerative colitis. Stomach Intestine. 2008;43:1935–46. (in Japanese)
4. Tanabe H, Iwashita A. Pathological diagnosis of ulcerative colitis-associated colorectal tumors update. Intestine. 2018;22:7–17. (in Japanese)

Development and Course of Inflammatory Bowel Disease-Associated Intestinal Cancer

Takashi Hisabe

In recent years, due to the increase in the number of patients with inflammatory bowel disease (IBD) and the prolonged duration of the disease, countermeasures against IBD-associated intestinal cancer have become increasingly important. The frequency of ulcerative colitis-associated colorectal cancer (UCAC) is significantly higher than that of the general population [1], and surveillance colonoscopy is recommended for early detection [2–4]. It has been reported to contribute to the reduction of colorectal cancer incidence and mortality [5]. However, early detection of UCAC is often difficult because the boundary between the tumor and the surrounding mucosa is unclear due to modification by chronic inflammation, and because the tumor develops in a bottom-up fashion from the deep glands to the middle layer of the glandular duct, resulting in little change in the mucosal alterations.

The development, growth, and progression of sporadic colorectal cancer (CRC) have been investigated by various methods. Molecular biological studies have pointed out genetic abnormalities, and the adenoma-carcinoma sequence theory [6], de novo carcinoma theory [7], and serrated pathway theory [8] have been proposed as the carcinogenic mechanism in sporadic colorectal cancer. In contrast, the dysplasia-carcinoma sequence theory has been proposed as the mechanism of IBD-associated carcinogenesis. *TP53* mutation is highly prevalent in UC [9, 10], but the *APC* and *KRAS* are not involved [11, 12]. In addition, abnormalities in mismatch repair genes and CpG island methylation [13–15] have been found in early stages of the disease, leading from low-grade dysplasia to high-grade dysplasia and then to carcinoma.

Clinical studies have been performed to retrospectively find morphological changes and to clarify the initial appearance of sporadic colorectal cancer using enteral radiographs and endoscopic images [16–18]. However, there have been few retrospective studies of IBD-associated intestinal cancer based on such imaging findings. We conducted a nationwide questionnaire survey [19] on endoscopic findings within 3 years of UCAC detection. The findings of 54 lesions in 49 cases are summarized as follows; approximately 40% of the initial lesions of UCAC were endoscopically visible as localized lesions, while the remaining 60% were judged to be inflammatory mucosal lesions. For 73.6% of advanced cancer, the initial lesion underwent rapid growth and became advanced cancer within 3 years; they accounted for 25.9% of the total cancers. Furthermore, we found that white light colonoscopy images obtained within 2 years before the diagnosis of UCAC were retrospectively reviewed at our hospital [20]. Of the 27 UCAC lesions (11 early stage; 16 advanced stage), 25.9% were initially visible and 74.1% were invisible. Invisible lesions were more common in the rectum and in patients with inflammation and left-sided colitis.

Wang et al. [21] examined the rate of early cancers missed surveillance of elderly patients with IBD. They presumed that the lesions missed by colonoscopy within 36 months of cancer detection were 15.1% in Crohn's disease (CD) and 15.8% in UC. Rutter et al. [22] performed surveillance endoscopy every 1–2 years in 600 patients with UC and reported that 30 (5%) colorectal cancers occurred. Sixteen of the 30 patients had interval cancer, which was not detected by endoscopy prior to cancer detection. Of these, 13 were found to have advanced cancer. Thus, in the past, IBD-associated intestinal cancer was difficult to detect at an early stage and was often detected as advanced cancer. Time-trend analysis revealed that the incidence rate of advanced CRC and interval CRC has steadily decreased over the past four decades. The incidence of dysplasia has increased, presumably due to the recent use of chromoendoscopy that was twice more effective at detecting dysplasia compared with white light endoscopy. In recent years, improvements in endoscopic image quality and the combination of image-enhanced endoscopy have made it possible to detect dysplasia and cancer at an early stage [23, 24].

T. Hisabe (✉)
Department of Gastroenterology, Fukuoka University Chikushi Hospital, Chikushino, Japan
e-mail: hisabe@cis.fukuoka-u.ac.jp

T. Matsui et al. (eds.), *Atlas of Inflammatory Bowel Disease-Associated Intestinal Cancer*,
https://doi.org/10.1007/978-981-19-3413-1_5

In addition, a Japanese RCT [25] comparing random biopsy and targeted biopsy in surveillance endoscopy reported that the number of tumors detected per endoscopy was not significantly different between random biopsy (0.168) and targeted biopsy (0.211). In recent years, targeted biopsy with chromoendoscopy has become the mainstream for surveillance because it is considered to be more efficient and cost-effective. On the other hand, there is a report [26] that 12.8% of lesions found by chromoendoscopic surveillance for UC and CD were found by random biopsy. It is important to keep in mind that there are still a few lesions that are not visible from retrospective studies.

The relative risk of small bowel cancer and colorectal cancer in CD is reported to be 31.2 (95% CI: 15.9–60.9) and 2.5 (95% CI: 1.3–4.7), respectively [27], and the cumulative incidence of colorectal cancer was reported to be 2.9% at 10 years, 5.6% at 20 years, and 8.3% at 30 years. In our study [28], the relative risk of colorectal cancer was similar, 3.2 (95% CI: 1.2–6.9), but the cumulative incidence was lower, 0.25% at 10 years and 0.58% at 20 years. Unlike in Europe and the US, where right-sided colon cancer is more common, anal canal cancer and rectal cancer are more common in Japan [29]. In CD, endoscopic surveillance is often difficult due to the presence of anal lesions and intestinal stenosis, and the cancer is often detected as advanced stage cancer. In our hospital, rectal biopsy by colonoscopy or biopsy of the rectum under anesthesia is performed for patients with anorectal disease for more than 10 years as surveillance for CD. Five (4.9%) of 103 patients with asymptomatic patients were found to have anorectal cancer [30].

The natural history of CD-associated cancers of the gastrointestinal tract has rarely been examined by analyzing imaging findings. At this time, the pathway of cancer progression cannot be estimated.

1 A Retrospective Study of UC-Associated Cancer

1.1 Early Stage Cancer

Case 1: Presumed neoplastic lesion retrospectively 30s, male

Extensive colitis, Chronic continuous type, disease duration 10 years

In 200X-10, he was diagnosed with UC of extensive colitis type and was treated with 5-aminosalicyclic acid (5-ASA) and steroids.

The patient was treated with biologics for steroid dependence in 200X-5.

A total colonoscopy performed in 200X showed a 15-mm superficial elevated type lesion of irregularity with a central white exudate in the sigmoid colon. Narrow-band imaging (NBI) with magnifying endoscopy (ME) of the edge of the lesion showed that the vessel pattern and surface pattern were both irregular and JNET classification type 2B (Fig. 1a–c). Histopathological findings were well to moderately differentiated adenocarcinoma, pTis.

Retrospective review of endoscopic findings

Twenty-four months prior to the diagnosis of cancer: the background mucosa was mildly active, and a granular superficial elevated type lesion (white arrow) was found in the sigmoid colon, which was diagnosed as tubular adenoma on biopsy, and an erythematous reddened inflammatory polyp was found on the left side of the same area (Fig. 2a).

Fourteen months prior to cancer diagnosis: the background mucosa was mildly active, with no change in the morphology of the granular flat type lesion of the sigmoid colon (white arrow). A retrospective review of the endoscopic images revealed a pale erythematous area with white

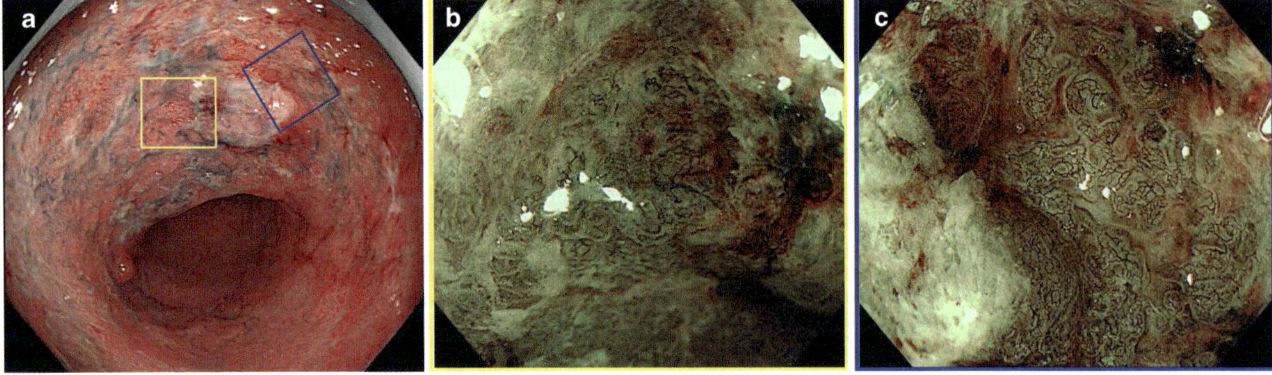

Fig. 1 (**a**) White light observation reveals a 15-mm in size superficial elevated type with indistinct borders and white moss. (**b** and **c**) NBI with ME shows irregular findings in the vessel pattern and surface pattern

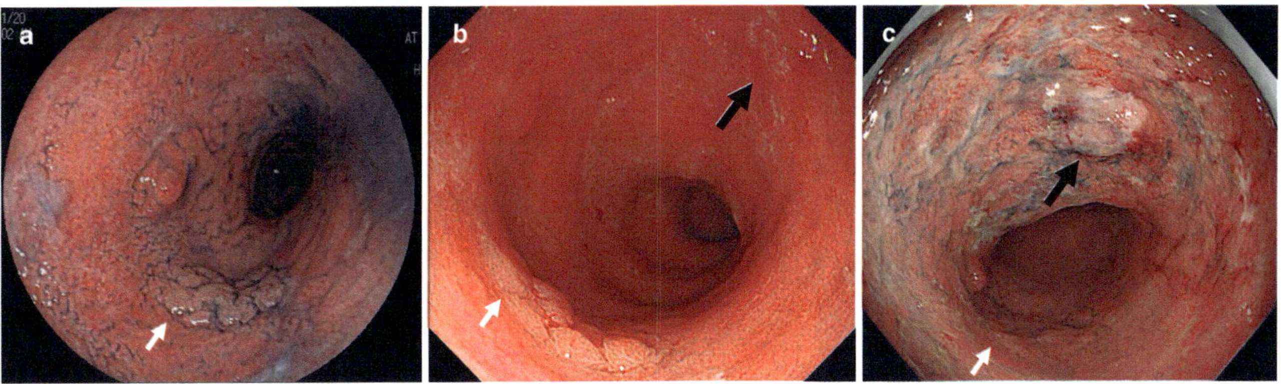

Fig. 2 (**a**) 24 months before cancer diagnosis. (**b**) 14 months before cancer diagnosis. (**c**) At the time of cancer diagnosis

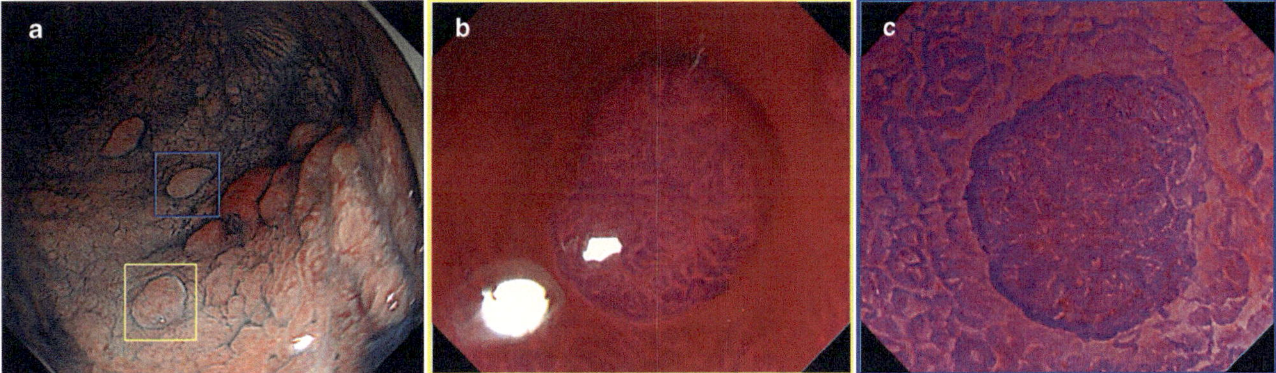

Fig. 3 (**a**) On white light observation, a well-defined superficial elevated type lesion of approximately 2 mm in size is seen around an intensely erythematous inflammatory polyp. (**b** and **c**) Pit pattern observation shows findings of V_I-low irregularity pattern

exudate on the contralateral side of this flat type lesion (black arrow) (Fig. 2b).

At the time of carcinoma diagnosis: the background mucosa was in a mildly active stage, and the pale erythematous area with flat elevation (white arrow) contralateral white exudate was enlarged and seen as a low superficial elevated type lesion with indistinct and irregular borders (black arrow) (Fig. 2c).

Case 2: A case in which no neoplastic lesion is presumed retrospectively
30s, male

Left-sided colitis, Chronic continuous type, disease duration 14 years

He was diagnosed as UC with left-sided colitis type in 200X-14 and treated with 5-ASA and steroids.

A total colonoscopy performed in 200X revealed a superficial elevated type lesion with a well-defined round shape of about 2 mm around an inflammatory polyp with intense redness of Rb. Pit pattern analysis by magnifying chromoendoscopy of two of these elevated lesions showed a V_I-low irregularity pattern (Fig. 3a–c). Histopathological findings showed that lesion presented in Fig. 3b was well-differentiated adenocarcinoma, pTis, and lesion presented in Fig. 3c was severe dysplasia with dysplasia in the other part of the surrounding mucosa.

Retrospective review of endoscopic findings

Twenty-four months before the diagnosis of cancer: the background mucosa was mildly active, with a strongly erythematous, analogous, raised lesion (white arrow) on Rb and a pale erythematous area on its antral side (Fig. 4a).

Thirteen months prior to cancer diagnosis: background mucosa was mildly active, with intensely erythematous raised lesions (white arrows) on the anal side. Biopsy of the same area showed mild to moderate active inflammation (Fig. 4b).

At the time of carcinoma diagnosis: the background mucosa was mildly active, with an intensely erythematous raised lesion (white arrow) with a well-defined superficial elevated type (black arrow) on the anal side (Fig. 4c).

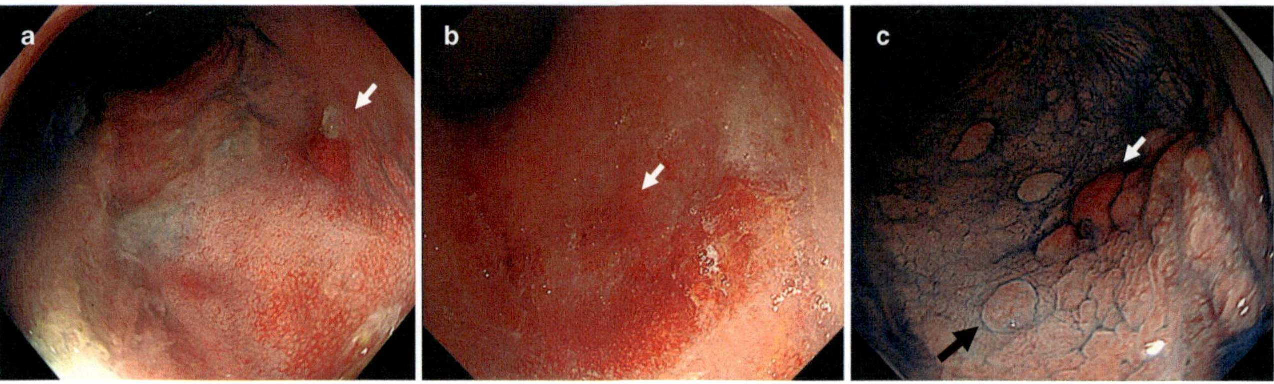

Fig. 4 (**a**) 24 months before cancer diagnosis. (**b**) 13 months before cancer diagnosis. (**c**) At the time of cancer diagnosis

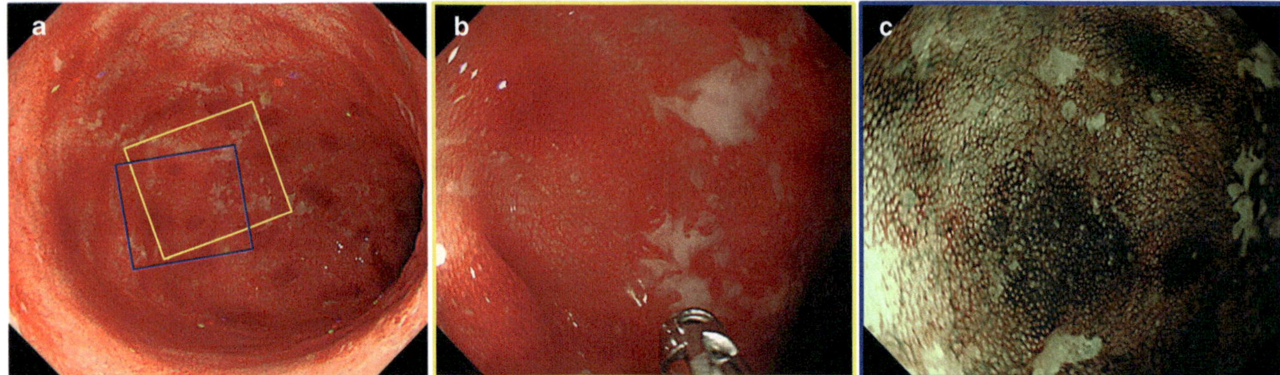

Fig. 5 (**a**) White light observation reveals multiple erythematous plaques and erosions. (**b** and **c**) NBI with ME shows regular findings of vessel pattern and surface pattern

Case 3: A case in which no neoplastic lesion is presumed retrospectively
40s, male

Left-sided colitis, relapse-remitting type, disease duration 13 years

In 200X-13, he was diagnosed as UC of left-sided colitis type and treated with 5-ASA and steroids.

The patient was treated with biologics for steroid dependence in 200X-5.

A total colonoscopy performed in 200X showed multiple erythematous plaques and erosions in the sigmoid colon, and NBI with ME showed that the vessel pattern and surface pattern were both regular with no obvious neoplastic changes, which was a JNET classification type 1 (Fig. 5a–c). Histopathological findings were well-differentiated adenocarcinoma, pTis.

Retrospective review of endoscopic findings

Twenty-nine months before cancer diagnosis: The background mucosa was mildly active, with multiple erythematous plaques in the sigmoid colon (Fig. 6a).

At the time of cancer diagnosis: the background mucosa was mildly active, with multiple erythematous plaques and erosions (black arrow) in the sigmoid colon (Fig. 6b).

1.2 Advanced Cancer

Case 4: A case in which no neoplastic lesion is presumed retrospectively
30s, male

Extensive colitis, Chronic continuous type, disease duration 19 years

On 200X-19, he was diagnosed with UC of extensive colitis type and treated with steroids and 5-ASA.

Total colonoscopy performed in 200X showed a narrowed lumen with ulcer scars in the sigmoid colon and an irregular depressed lesion with a circumferential ulceration on its anal side. NBI with ME showed that the vessel pattern was an avascular area with thick, tortuous vessels, and the surface pattern was indistinct, which was a JNET classification type 3 (Fig. 7a–c). Histopathological findings showed well-differentiated adenocarcinoma, pT2, and dysplasia in the surrounding mucosa.

Retrospective review of endoscopic findings

Twelve months before cancer diagnosis: the background mucosa was at the remission stage and showed narrowing of the lumen with multiple ulcer scars (Fig. 8a).

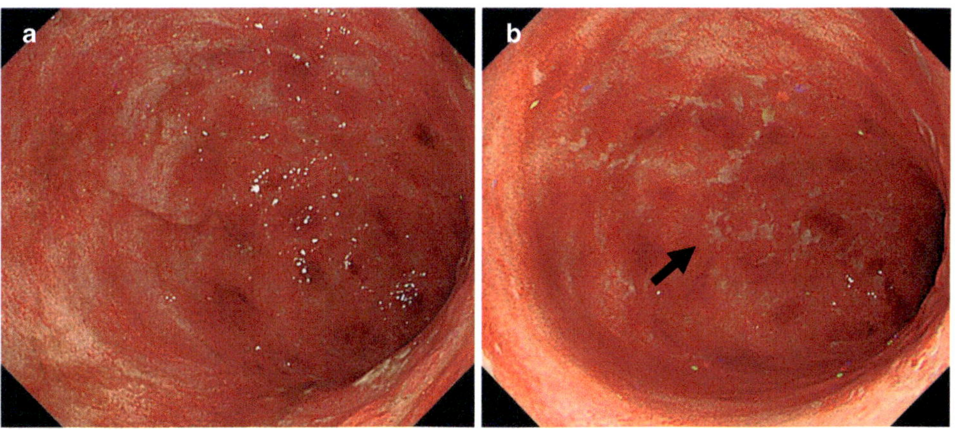

Fig. 6 (**a**) 29 months before cancer diagnosis. (**b**) At the time of cancer diagnosis

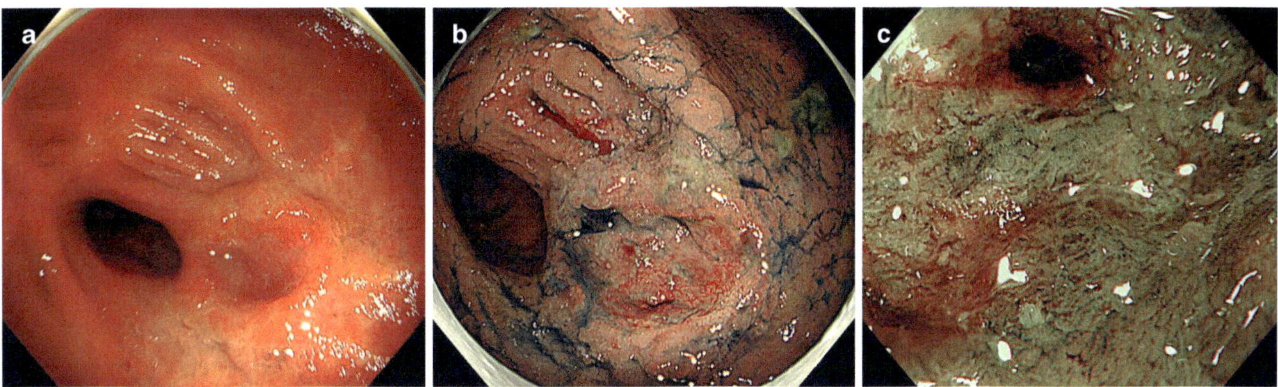

Fig. 7 (**a** and **b**) White light observation shows a narrowing of the lumen with an ulcer scar and an irregular depressed lesion with a circumferential crest on its anal side. (**c**) On NBI with ME, the vessel pattern shows an avascular area with thick, tortuous vessels, and the surface pattern is indistinct, with JNET classification type 3

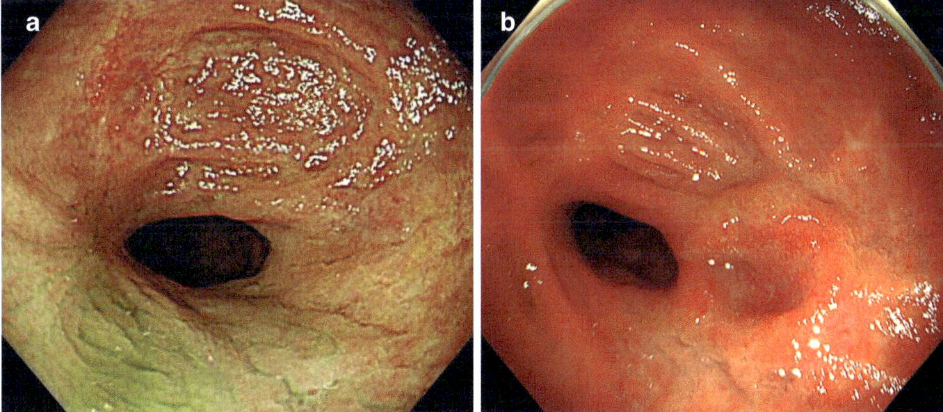

Fig. 8 (**a**) 12 months before cancer diagnosis. (**b**) At the time of cancer diagnosis

At the time of cancer diagnosis: the background mucosa was at the remission stage and showed an irregular depressed lesion with a circumferential ulceration on the anal side of the narrow area (Fig. 8b).

Case 5: A case in which no neoplastic lesion is presumed retrospectively
30s, male

Extensive colitis, relapse-remitting type, disease duration 14 years

In 200X-14, he was diagnosed with UC of extensive colitis type and was treated with 5-ASA and steroids.

A total colonoscopy performed in 200X showed a circumferential stenosis of the descending colon, with a vessel pattern of irregular and a surface pattern of absent on NBI with ME, which was a JENT classification type 3. The pit pattern analysis showed a V_I-high irregularity pattern (Fig. 9a–c).

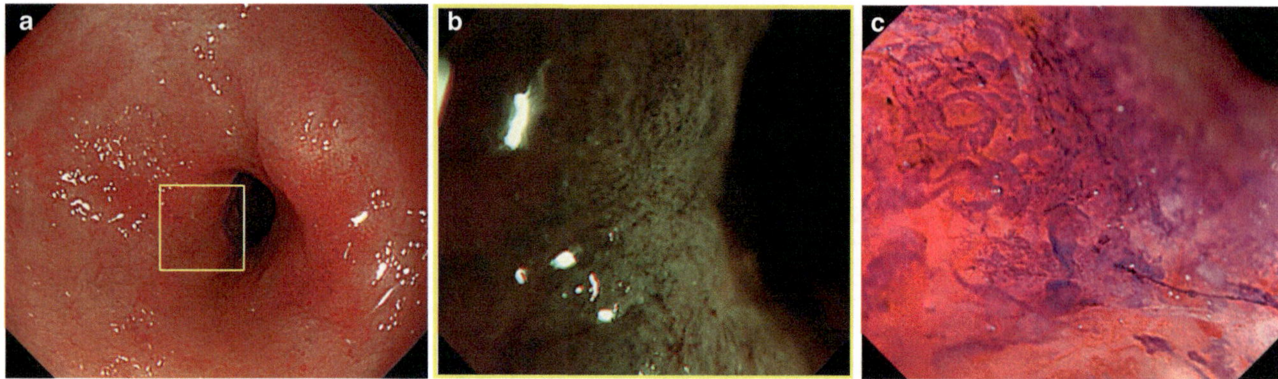

Fig. 9 (**a**) White light observation showed a circumferential stenosis. (**b** and **c**) NBI with ME showed an irregular vessel pattern and an absent surface pattern, and pit pattern observation showed a V_I-high irregularity pattern

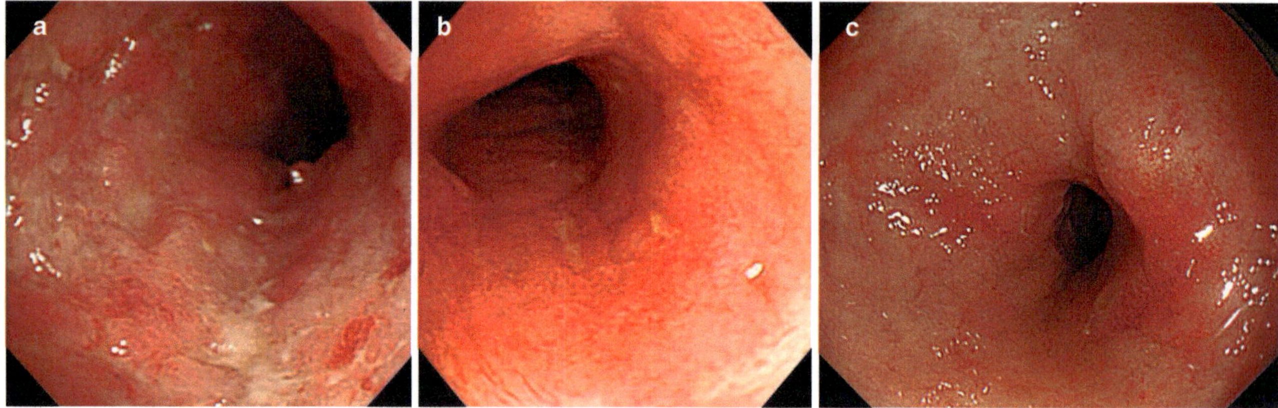

Fig. 10 (**a**) 76 months before cancer diagnosis. (**b**) 39 months before cancer diagnosis. (**c**) At the time of cancer diagnosis

Histopathological findings were very well to well-differentiated adenocarcinoma, pT4.

Retrospective review of endoscopic findings

Seventy-six months prior to cancer diagnosis: the background mucosa was moderately active, with generalized ulceration of the descending colon (Fig. 10a).

Thirty-nine months prior to cancer diagnosis: the background mucosa was in remission and showed a slight narrowing of the lumen (Fig. 10b).

At the time of cancer diagnosis: the background mucosa was in a mildly active stage, with a circumfrential stenosis (Fig. 10c).

2 A Retrospective Study of CD-Associated Cancer

2.1 Advanced Cancer

Case 6: A case in which neoplastic lesion is presumed retrospectively
30s, female

Ileocolonic type CD, disease duration 13 years

In 199X-13, the patient was found to have a perianal fistula and was diagnosed with ileocolonic type CD and was treated with nutritional therapy and 5-ASA.

The patient was treated with biological agents for worsening of symptoms in 199X-3.

A biopsy of the mucosa of the anal canal during drainage by the Seaton method in 199X-2 revealed atypical epithelium, which was observed endoscopically every few months thereafter.

A total colonoscopy performed in 199X showed active lesions in the descending colon and rectum, including an irregular ulcer on the Rb and a low, raised lesion with superficial granular and villous indistinct margins over the entire lumen, which was biopsied as a very well-differentiated adenocarcinoma (Fig. 11). A perineal rectal amputation was performed, and the histopathological findings were very well to well-differentiated adenocarcinoma with extracellular mucinous degeneration, pT3.

Retrospective review of endoscopic findings

Nine months before cancer diagnosis: the rectum was slightly narrowed and showed ulcers with white exudate (Fig. 12a).

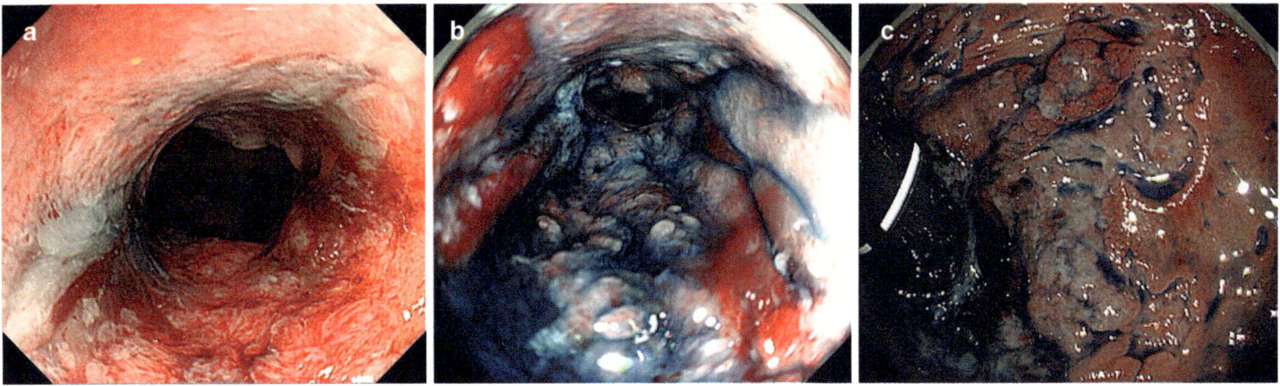

Fig. 11 (**a** and **b**) White light observation revealed a low, raised lesion of indistinct length with superficial granular and villous borders over the entire lumen. (**c**) Retroflexion view showed an irregular ulcer on the oral side of the dentate line

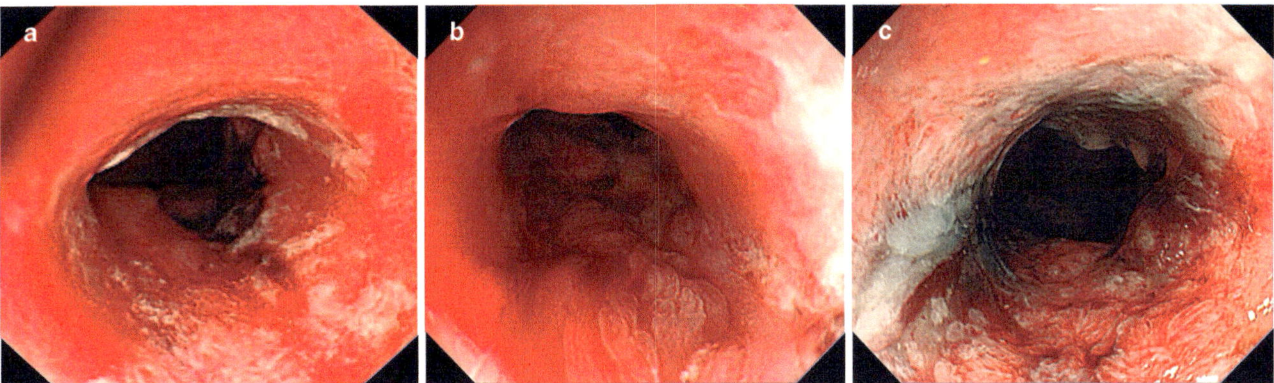

Fig. 12 (**a**) 9 months before cancer diagnosis. (**b**) 3 months before cancer diagnosis. (**c**) At the time of cancer diagnosis

Three months before cancer diagnosis: villous protuberant lesions were noted (Fig. 12b).

At the time of carcinoma diagnosis: A low, raised lesion with indistinct borders was noted (Fig. 12c).

Case 7: A case in which neoplastic lesion is presented retrospectively
50s, female

Colonic type CD, disease duration 25 years

He was diagnosed with colonic CD in 199X-25 and treated with 5-ASA.

She was treated with biological agents for worsening of symptoms in 199X-5.

In 199X, she had right lower quadrant abdominal pain and underwent a total colonoscopy, which revealed a narrowed ascending colon with an irregular depressed lesion with a circumferential ulceration (Fig. 13). She was diagnosed with colorectal cancer and underwent right hemicolectomy, and the histopathological findings were poorly differentiated adenocarcinoma with intra- and extracellular mucinous degeneration, pT4.

Retrospective review of endoscopic findings

Thirty-six months prior to cancer diagnosis: a club-shaped and sessile type inflammatory polyp was found in the ascending colon (Fig. 14a), with a sea anemone and a club-shaped inflammatory polyp on its anal side (Fig. 14b).

At the time of cancer diagnosis: Type 2 advanced cancer was found in the ascending colon. Club-shaped and sessile type inflammatory polyps, considered to be the same lesions as in Fig. 14a, were seen, but the sea anemone and club-shaped polyps could not be identified, and colorectal cancer was found in the same area (Fig. 14c).

Fig. 13 (**a**) White light observation revealed an irregular depressed lesion with a circumferential crest. (**b** and **c**) Inflammatory polyps are present on the oral side of the lesion

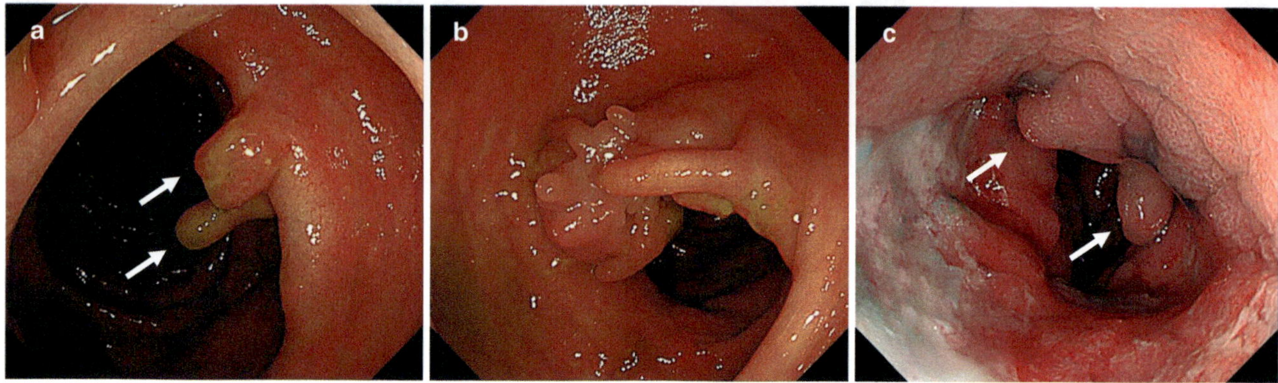

Fig. 14 (**a** and **b**) 36 months before cancer diagnosis. (**c**) At the time of cancer diagnosis

References

1. Jess T, Rungoe C, Peyrin-Biroulet L. Risk of colorectal cancer in patients with ulcerative colitis: a meta-analysis of population-based cohort studies. Clin Gastroenterol Hepatol. 2012;10:639–45.
2. Cairns SR, Scholefield JH, Dunlop MG, et al. Guidelines for colorectal cancers screening and surveillance in moderate and high risk groups (update from 2002). Gut. 2010;59:666–89.
3. Magro F, Gionchetti P, Eliakim R, et al. Third European evidence-based consensus on diagnosis and management of ulcerative colitis: part 1: definitions, diagnosis, extra-intestinal manifestations, pregnancy, cancer surveillance, surgery, and ileo-anal pouch disorders. J Crohns Colitis. 2017;11:649–70.
4. Rubin DT, Ananthakrishnan AN, Siegel CA, et al. ACG clinical guideline: ulcerative colitis in adults. Am J Gastroenterol. 2019;114:384–413.
5. Bye WA, Ma C, Nguyen TM, et al. Strategies for detecting colorectal cancer in patients with inflammatory bowel disease: a Cochrane systematic review and meta-analysis. Am J Gastroenterol. 2018;113:1801–9.
6. Vogelstein B, Fearon ER, Hamilton SR, et al. Genetic alterations during colorectal tumor development. N Engl J Med. 1988;319:525–32.
7. Spratt JS Jr, Ackerman LV. Small primary adenocarcinomas of the colon and rectum. JAMA. 1962;179:337–46.
8. Leggett B, Whitehall V. Role of the serrated pathway in colorectal cancer pathogenesis. Gastroenterology. 2010;138:2088–100.
9. Hussain SP, Amstad P, Raja K, et al. Increased p53 mutation load in noncancerous colon tissue from ulcerative colitis: a cancer-prone chronic. Cancer Res. 2000;60:3333–7.
10. Brentnall TA, Crispin DA, Rabinovitch PS, et al. Mutations in the p53 gene: an early marker of neoplastic progression in ulcerative colitis. Gastroenterology. 1994;107:369–78.
11. Maia L, Dinis J, Bravo M, et al. Who takes the lead in the development of ulcerative colitis-associated colorectal cancers: mutator, suppressor, or methylator pathway? Cancer Genet Cytogenet. 2005;162:68–73.
12. Burmer GC, Levine DS, Kulander BG, et al. c-Ki-ras mutations in chronic ulcerative colitis and sporadic colon carcinoma. Gastroenterology. 1990;99:416–20.
13. Chiba T, Marusawa H, Ushijima T. Inflammation-associated cancer development in digestive organs: mechanisms and roles for genetic and epigenetic modulation. Gastroenterology. 2012;143:550–63.
14. Fujii S, Tominaga K, Kitajima K, et al. Methylation of the oestrogen receptor gene in non-neoplastic epithelium as a marker of colorectal neoplasia risk in longstanding and extensive ulcerative colitis. Gut. 2005;54:1287–92.
15. Toiyama Y, Okugawa Y, Tanaka K, et al. A panel of methylated microRNA biomarkers for identifying high-risk patients with ulcerative colitis-associated colorectal cancer. Gastroenterology. 2017;153:1634–46.

16. Watari J, Saitoh Y, Obara T, et al. Natural history of colorectal nonpolypoid adenomas: a prospective colonoscopic study and relation with cell. Am J Gastroenterol. 2002;97:2109–15.
17. Hisabe T, Tsuda S, Matsui T, Iwashita A. Natural history of small colorectal protuberant adenomas. Dig Endosc. 2010;22(Suppl 1):43–6.
18. Hisabe T, Hirai F, Matsui T. Development and progression of colorectal cancer based on follow-up analysis. Dig Endosc. 2014;26(Suppl 2):73–7.
19. Yamasaki K, Matsui T, Hisabe T, et al. Retrospective analysis of the growth speed of 54 lesions of colitis-associated colorectal neoplasia. Anticancer Res. 2016;36:3731–40.
20. Hisabe T, Matsui T, Yamasaki K, et al. Possible earlier diagnosis of ulcerative colitis-associated neoplasia: a retrospective analysis of interval cases during surveillance. J Clin Med. 2021;10:1927.
21. Wang YR, Cangemi JR, Loftus E, et al. Rate of early/missed colorectal cancers after colonoscopy in older patients with or without inflammatory bowel disease in the United States. Am J Gastroenterol. 2013;108:444–9.
22. Rutter M, Saunders B, Wilkinson K, et al. Thirty-year analysis of a colonoscopic surveillance program for neoplasia in ulcerative colitis. Gastroenterology. 2006;130:1030–8.
23. Bessissow T, Dulai PS, Restellini S, et al. Comparison of endoscopic dysplasia detection techniques in patients with ulcerative colitis: a systematic review and network meta-analysis. Inflamm Bowel Dis. 2018;24:2518–26.
24. Feuerstein JD, Rakowsky S, Sattler L, et al. Meta-analysis of dye-based chromoendoscopy compared with standard- and high-definition white light endoscopy in patients with inflammatory bowel disease at increased risk of colon cancer. Gastrointest Endosc. 2019;90:186–95.
25. Watanabe T, Ajioka Y, Mitsuyama K, et al. Comparison of targeted vs random biopsies for surveillance of ulcerative colitis-associated colorectal. Gastroenterology. 2016;151:1122–30.
26. Moussata D, Allez M, Cazala-Hatem D, et al. Are random biopsies still useful for the detection of neoplasia in patients with IBD undergoing surveillance colonoscopy with chromoendoscopy? Gut. 2018;67:616–24.
27. Canavan C, Abrams KR, Mayberry J. Meta-analysis: colorectal and small bowel cancer risk patients with Crohn's disease. Aliment Pharmacol Ther. 2006;23:1097–104.
28. Yano Y, Matsui T, Uno H, et al. Risks and clinical features of colorectal cancer complicating Crohn's disease in Japanese patients. Gastroenterol Hepatol. 2008;23:1683–8.
29. Higashi D, Katsuno H, Takahashi K, et al. Current state of and problems related to cancer of the intestine tract associated with Crohn's. Anticancer Res. 2016;36:3761–6.
30. Hirano Y, Futami K, Higashi D, et al. Anorectal cancer surveillance in Crohn's disease. J Anus Rectum Colon. 2018;2:145–54.

Part II

Cases of UC Associated Cancers

Early Cancer: 9 Cases with Various Features

Takashi Hisabe, Hiroshi Tanabe, Keisuke Kawasaki, Makoto Eizuka, Tamotsu Sugai, and Takayuki Matsumoto

T. Hisabe (✉)
Department of Gastroenterology, Fukuoka University Chikushi Hospital, Chikushino, Japan
e-mail: hisabe@cis.fukuoka-u.ac.jp

H. Tanabe
Department of Pathology, Fukuoka University Chikushi Hospital, Chikushino, Japan

K. Kawasaki
Department of Gastroenterology, Iwate Medical University, Iwate, Japan

Department of Medicine and Clinical Science, Graduate School of Medical Sciences, Kyushu University, Fukuoka, Japan

M. Eizuka
Department of Gastroenterology, Iwate Medical University, Iwate, Japan

Department of Molecular Diagnostic Pathology, Iwate Medical University, Iwate, Japan

T. Sugai
Department of Molecular Diagnostic Pathology, Iwate Medical University, Iwate, Japan

T. Matsumoto
Department of Gastroenterology, Iwate Medical University, Iwate, Japan

T. Matsui et al. (eds.), *Atlas of Inflammatory Bowel Disease-Associated Intestinal Cancer*,
https://doi.org/10.1007/978-981-19-3413-1_6

1 Case 1: Early-Stage Cancer with Extensive Dysplasia

Takashi Hisabe and Hiroshi Tanabe

20s, male (11 years of illness)

Type of disease: Extensive colitis
Clinical course: Relapse-remitting type
Macroscopic type: Sessile type (indistinct border)

History of Present Illness

After the diagnosis of ulcerative colitis, the patient was treated with 5-ASA.

Four years after the onset of the disease, the patient had an exacerbation of symptoms and was treated with steroids and granulocyte adsorption apheresis, but had repeated relapses and remissions.

Eleven years after the onset of symptoms, the patient underwent colonoscopy, which revealed sessile type early-stage colorectal cancer in the sigmoid colon (Fig. 1), and total colorectal resection was performed (Fig. 2).

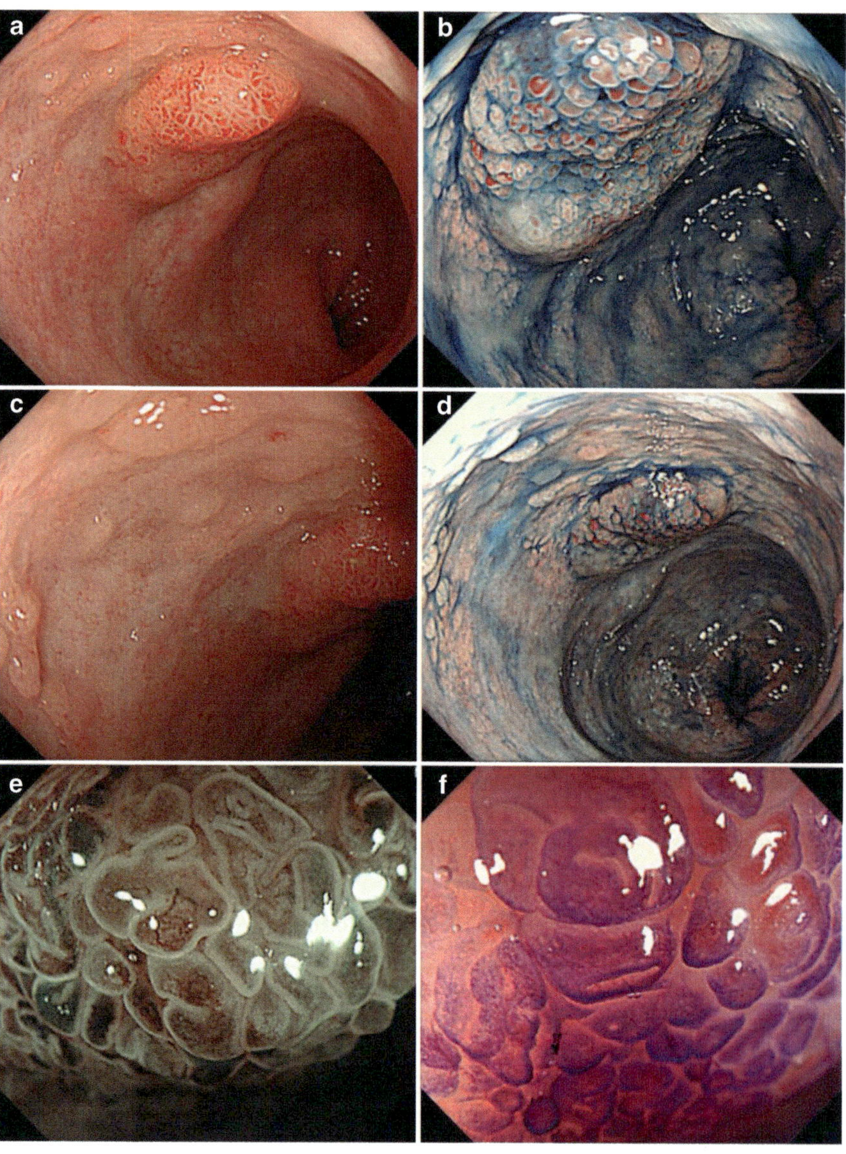

Fig. 1 Colonoscopic findings. (**a** and **b**) Conventional endoscopic observation showed an erythematous raised lesion in the sigmoid colon, and the border of the lesion was relatively clear after application of indigo carmine dye. (**c** and **d**) The surrounding background mucosa showed faded areas and granular mucosa. (**e**) NBI with magnified endoscopy (ME) showed that the vessel pattern was uniform in shape, symmetrical and regular in distribution and arrangement, and the surface pattern was regular with an arc-shaped epithelium at the marginal crypt epithelium, which was JNET classification type 2A. (**f**) The pit pattern showed type IV with a brain gyrus or villous pattern with no obvious irregular glandular structure

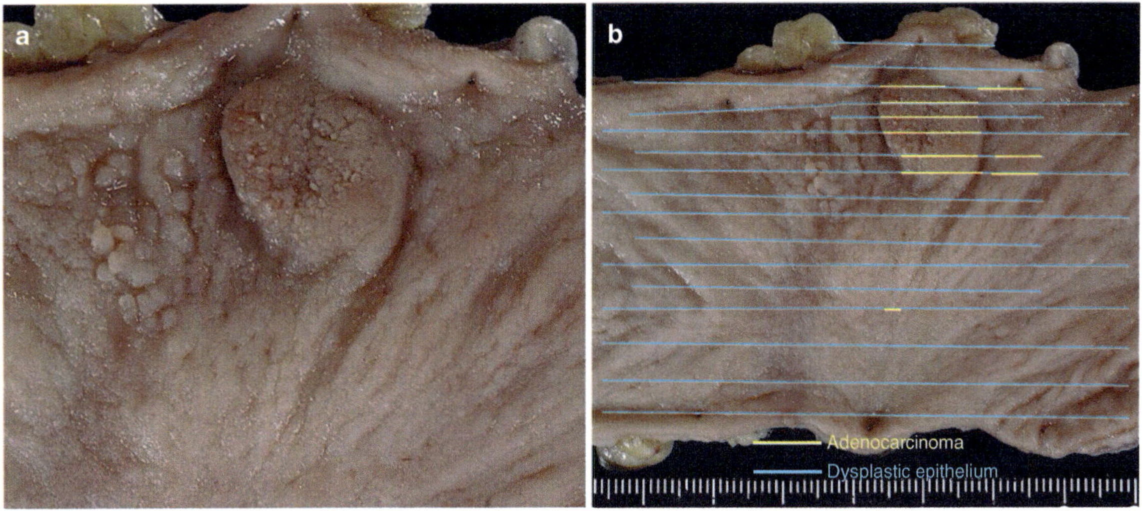

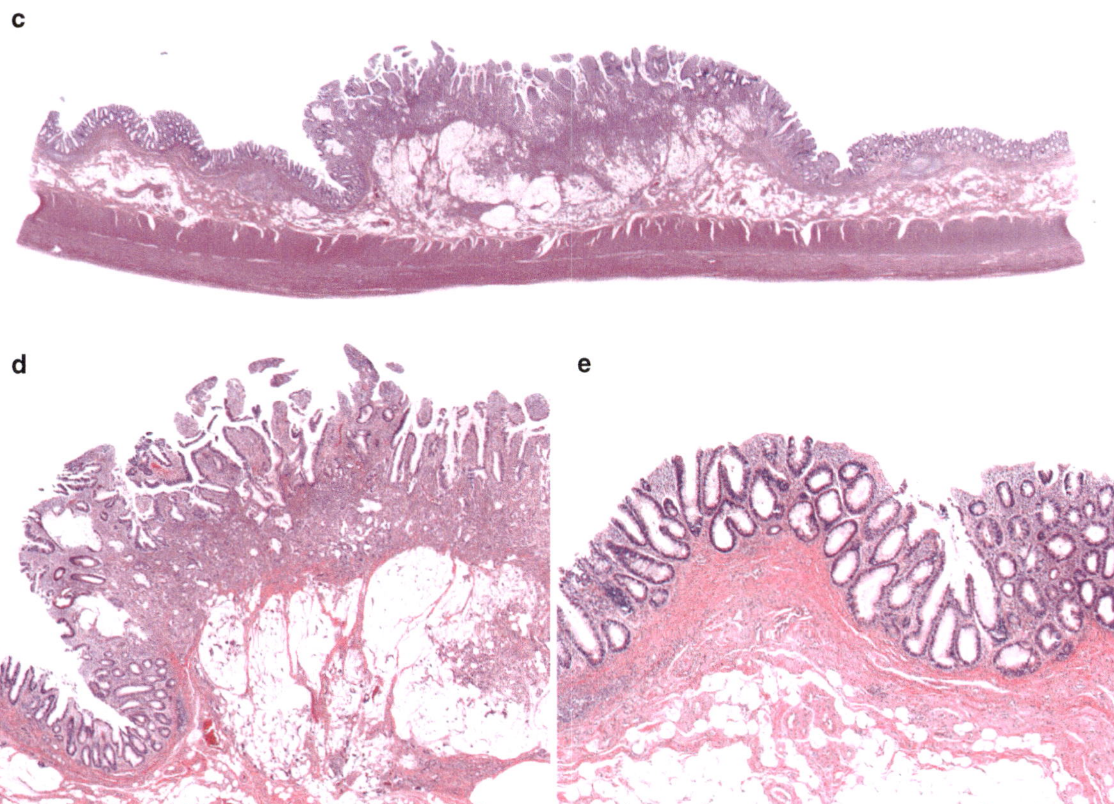

Fig. 2 Pathological image. (**a**) The resected specimen showed a 25 × 18 mm nodular irregular elevated lesion with granular changes on the anorectal side. (**b**) As shown in the reconstructed image, the nodular elevation was a carcinoma invading the submucosa (yellow line), surrounded by intramucosal carcinoma and dysplastic epithelium (yellow and blue line). (**c**) Lupe finding. The carcinoma had invaded the deeper portion of the submucosa with extracellular mucous degeneration. (**d**) Histopathologically, the superficial layer of the tumor at the nodular elevation was a very well-differentiated adenocarcinoma with a villous pattern (corresponding to endoscopic images Fig. 1e, f), and the deeper layer was a moderately to poorly differentiated adenocarcinoma with extracellular mucous degeneration. (**e**) Extensive dysplastic epithelium was seen in the surrounding mucosa

Pathological Diagnosis

- Sigmoid colon: Type 0-Is + IIb, 25 × 18 mm, very well to poorly differentiated adenocarcinoma with mucous degeneration, pT1b (SM, 2250 μm), Ly1b, V0, INF b, pPM0, pDM0, pN0.
- Stage I: pT1b, pN0, M0, P0, H0, R0, Cur A

Summary of the Case

Deeply elevated villous lesions with clear borders and relatively uniform shape were accompanied by extracellular mucous degeneration, and the extensive faded and granular mucosa around the elevated lesions was dysplasia.

2 Case 2: Early-Stage Cancer That Was Difficult to Distinguish from Sporadic Cancer at Preoperative Diagnosis

Takashi Hisabe and Hiroshi Tanabe

30s, male (17 years of illness)

Type of disease: Extensive colitis

Clinical course: Relapse-remitting type

Macroscopic type: Superficial elevated type (distinct border)

History of Present Illness

After the diagnosis of ulcerative colitis, he was treated with 5-ASA and azathioprine, and for the past several years.

The patient was maintained in remission.

Seventeen years after the onset of the disease, a surveillance colonoscopy was performed, which revealed early-stage colorectal cancer of superficial elevated type with well-defined borders in Ra (Fig. 3). Biopsy of the peri-tumor area showed no dysplasia, and the patient underwent endoscopic submucosal dissection for total biopsy (Fig. 4).

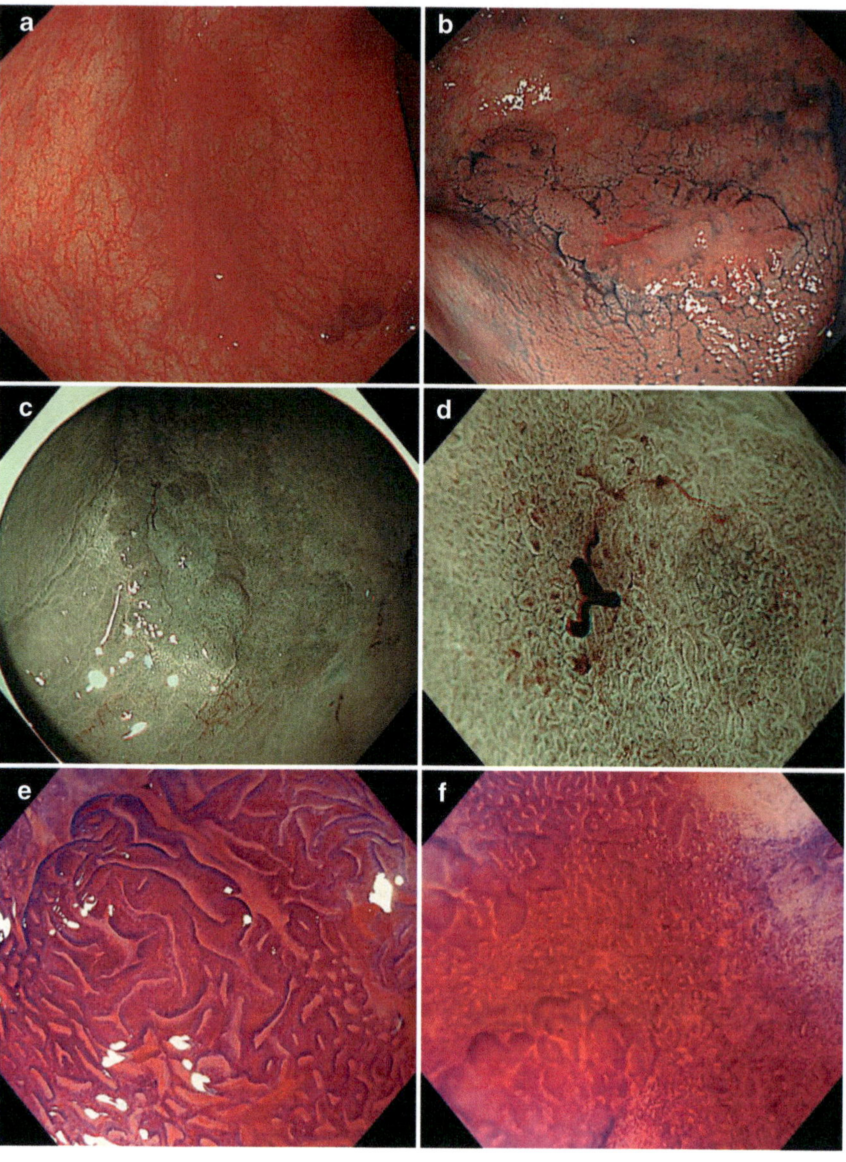

Fig. 3 Colonoscopic findings. (**a** and **b**) On conventional endoscopic observation, Ra showed an erythematous area with loss of vascular permeability, and after indigo carmine dye application, the lesion showed a superficial lesion with clear borders and pseudo-depression. (**c** and **d**) NBI endoscopy showed the lesion as brownish area and NBI with ME showed that the shape of the vessel pattern was relatively uniform and the distribution and arrangement were symmetrical and regular, while the surface pattern was generally regular, but some areas were indistinct and uneven in shape, which was JNET classification type 2B. (**e** and **f**) The tumor margin showed type IV and type III_L pit patterns, and the pseudoconcave showed small glandular ducts with uneven size and arrangement, and was diagnosed to be V_I-low irregularity

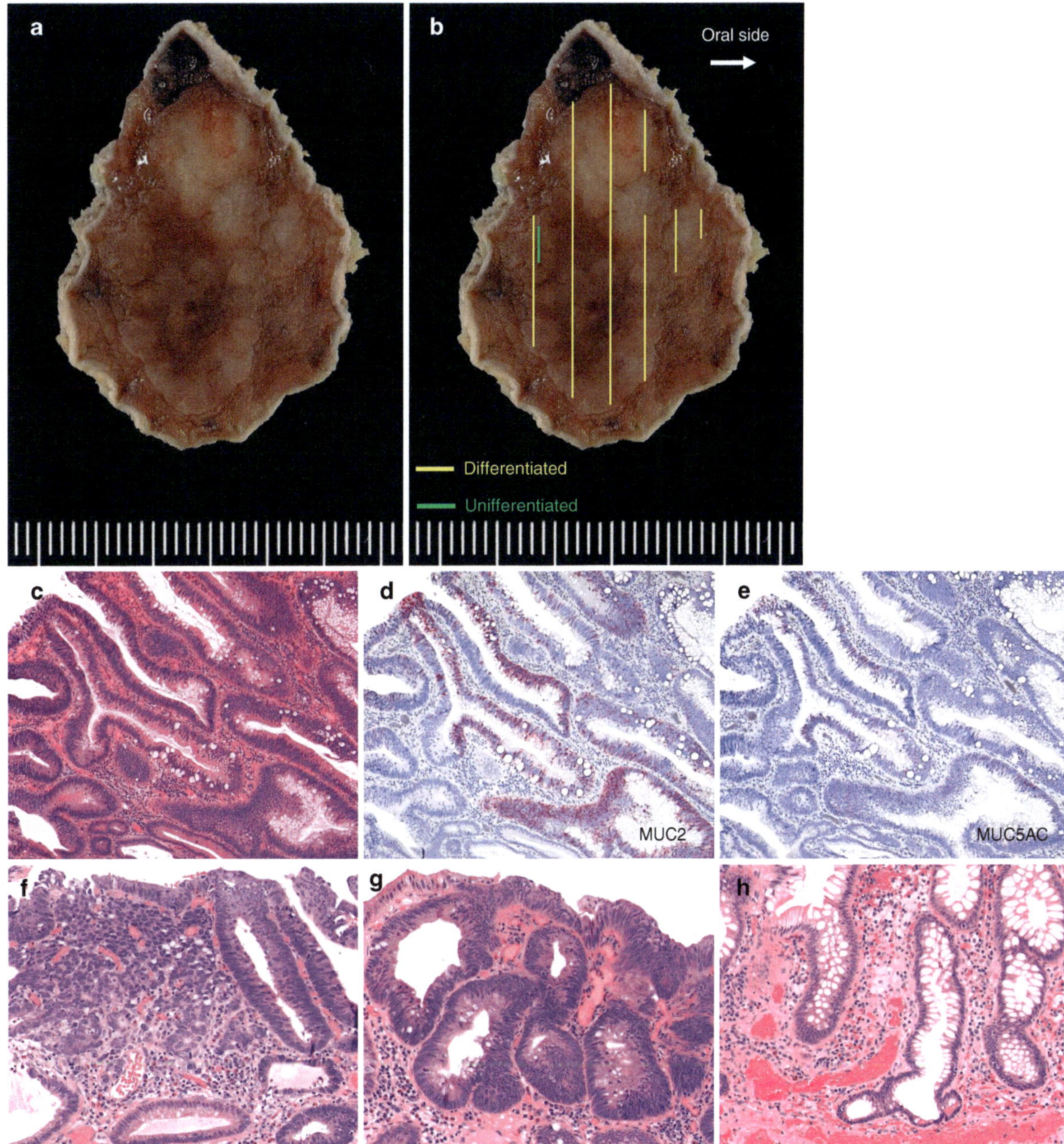

Fig. 4 Pathological image. (**a**) The resected specimen showed a 28 × 16 mm same color to faded flat-elevated lesion. (**b**) The lesion was mostly composed of very well to well-differentiated tubular adenocarcinoma (yellow line) and small area of poorly differentiated adenocarcinoma (green line). (**c**) Histopathological finding of very well to well-differentiated tubular adenocarcinoma. (**d** and **e**) Immunohistochemically, the tumor cells are positive for MUC2 (**d**) and CD10, and the mucin phenotype was predominantly intestinal type, but a small part was positive for MUC5AC (**e**), and mixed gastric phenotype was observed. Histologically, it is consistent with UC-associated cancer. (**f**) Small area of poorly differentiated adenocarcinoma was also seen on the anorectal side of the lesion. (**g**) The lesion had some borderless areas that were difficult to differentiate from adenoma. (**h**) The background mucosa was ulcerative colitis mucosa in remission stage with crypt distortion and Paneth cell metaplasia

Pathological Diagnosis

- Rectum (ESD): Type 0-IIa, 28 × 16 mm, very well to well-differentiated adenocarcinoma with focal adenomatous pattern and a small area of poor differentiation, pTis (M), Ly0, V0, INF a, pHM0, pVM0.

Summary of this Case

Sporadic early colorectal cancer was suspected because of the absence of surrounding dysplasia on endoscopic gross morphology and biopsy, but histopathologically it was UC-associated cancer.

3 Case 3: Early-Stage Cancer with Indistinct Borders

Takashi Hisabe and Hiroshi Tanabe

60s, male (disease duration: 27 years)

Type of disease: Extensive colitis

Clinical course: Chronic continuous type

Macroscopic type: flat type (indistinct border)

History of Present Illness

After the diagnosis of ulcerative colitis, the patient was treated with 5-ASA and steroids were administered in case of exacerbation.

Twenty-six years after the onset of the disease, his symptoms worsened and he was treated with steroids and azathioprine, but relapses occurred repeatedly.

Twenty-seven years after the onset of the disease, a colonoscopy was performed, and the sigmoid colon was found to have an indistinct flat type (Fig. 5).

The patient was found to have early-stage colorectal cancer and underwent a total colorectal resection (Fig. 6).

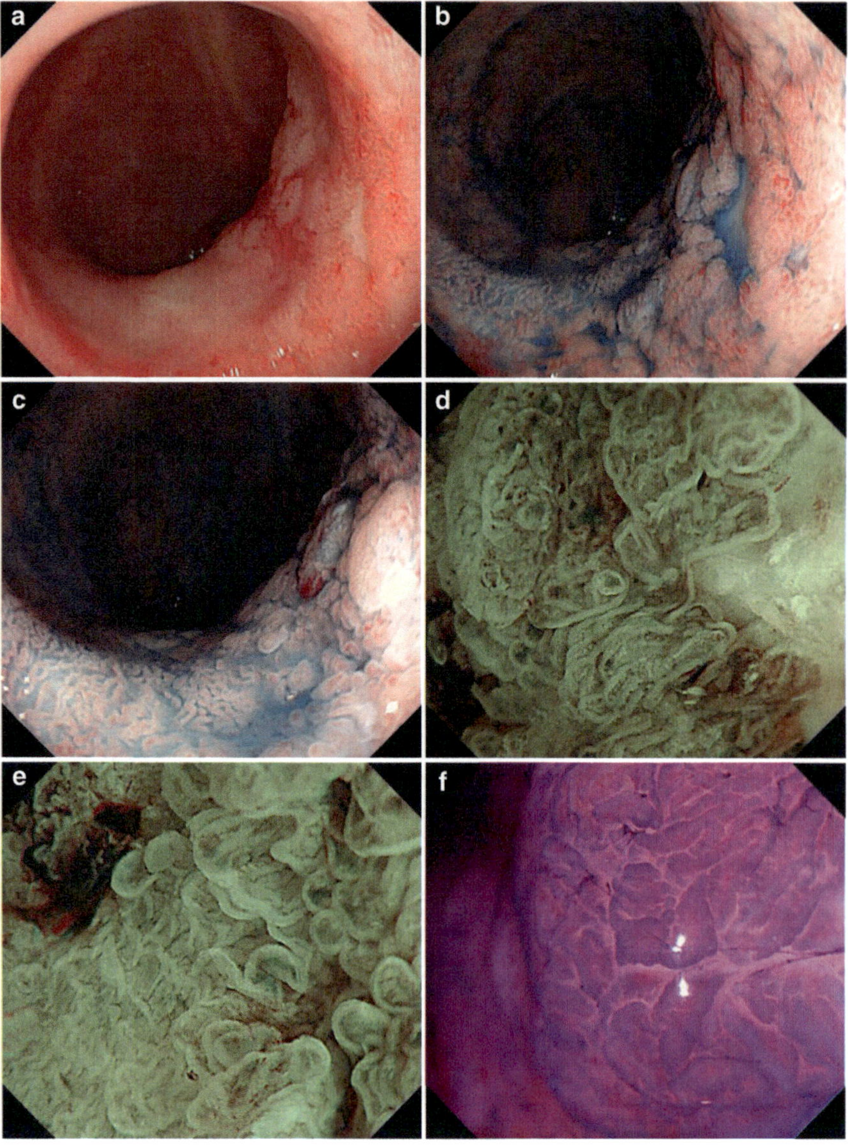

Fig. 5 Colonoscopic findings. (**a–c**) Conventional endoscopic observation revealed an erythematous area with erosions in the sigmoid colon. Chromoendoscopy showed a partly elevated lesion with unclear margin and villous surface. (**d** and **e**) NBI with ME showed that the vessel pattern was relatively uniform in shape and symmetrical in distribution and arrangement, and the surface pattern was regular with arcuate or papillary epithelium at the marginal crypt epithelium, which was a JNET classification type 2A. (**f**) The pit pattern showed type IV with a fern leaf-like villous pattern

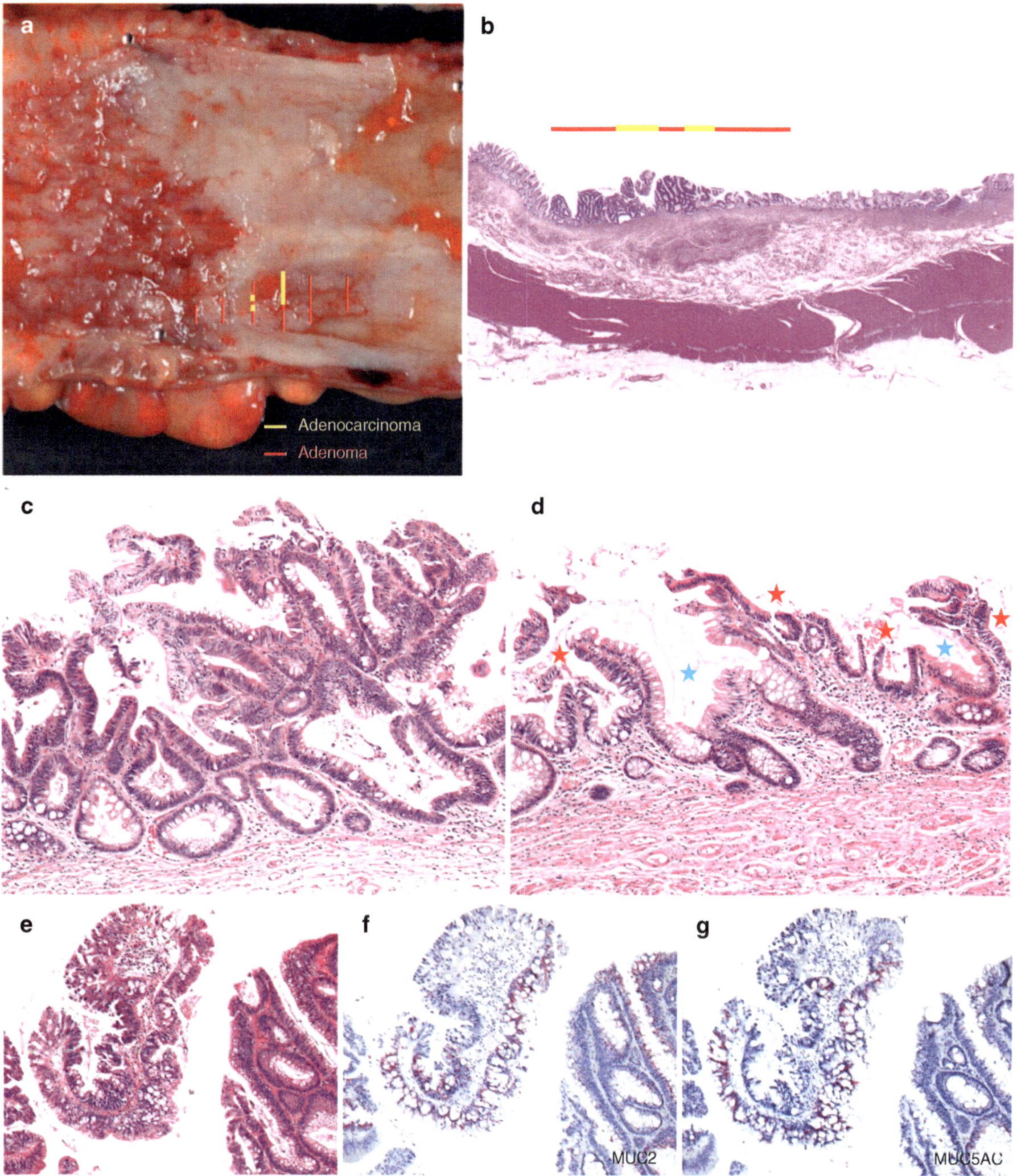

Fig. 6 Pathological image. (**a**) The resected specimen shows a 23 × 10 mm flat-elevated lesion. Grossly, the lesions are almost same color as the surrounding mucosa and have a granular to nodular surface. Adenocarcinoma was shown in yellow line and adenoma was shown in red line. (**b**) Lupe finding, there are multiple Ul-II ulcer scars due to ulcerative colitis in the background. (**c**–**e**) Histopathologically, well-differentiated tubular adenocarcinoma in the center of the tumor (**c**, **e**). At the tumor border, some tumor gland ducts (red star) and nontumor gland ducts (blue star) were mixed and gently transitioned, which made the border diagnosis difficult (**d**). (**f** and **g**) Immunohistochemically, the carcinoma area was positive for both MUC2 (**f**) and MUC5AC (**g**), and the mucin phenotype was mixed gastric and intestinal mucin phenotype, consistent with UC-associated carcinoma

Pathological Diagnosis

- Sigmoid colon: Type 0-IIa, 23 × 10 mm, well-differentiated adenocarcinoma in tubulovillous adenoma with moderate atypia, pTis (M), Ly0, V0, BD1, INF a, pPM0, pDM0, pN0.
- Stage 0: pTis, pN0, M0, P0, H0, R0, Cur A.

Summary of this Case

The tumor could be diagnosed by endoscopy, but the boundary with the surrounding mucosa was unclear due to the mixed tumor and nontumor tissue.

4 Case 4: Early-Stage Carcinoma of Sessile Type with Clear Borders

Takashi Hisabe and Hiroshi Tanabe

50s, female (25 years of illness)

Type of disease: left-sided colitis

Clinical course: Relapse-remitting type

Macroscopic type: Sessile type (distinct border)

History of Present Illness

After the diagnosis of ulcerative colitis, the patient was treated with 5-ASA, but he did not visit our hospital thereafter.

Twenty-five years after the diagnosis, upper abdominal pain and diarrhea appeared, and colonoscopy was performed. Multiple irregular elevated lesions were found in the colon, and the patient was diagnosed with colorectal cancer (Fig. 7) and underwent total colorectal resection (Fig. 8).

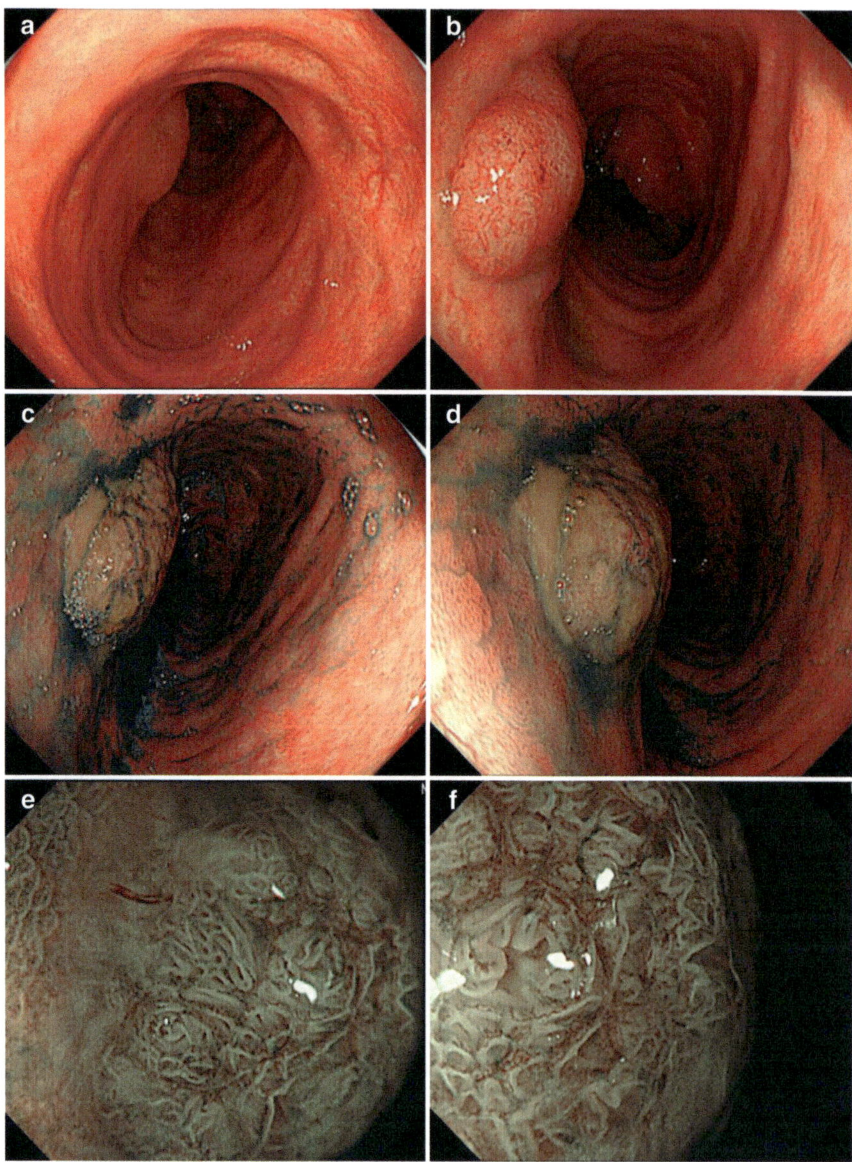

Fig. 7 Colonoscopic findings. (**a**–**d**) Conventional endoscopic observation showed an irregular hemispherical raised lesion of 15 mm in diameter with erythematous tone in the ascending colon, and chromoendoscopy showed the border of the lesion was relatively clear. The background mucosa had multiple ulcer scars, but no obvious neoplastic changes were noted. (**e** and **f**) NBI with ME showed that the vessel pattern was nonuniform shape, asymmetric and irregular in distribution and arrangement, and the surface pattern was regular, which was diagnosed to be a JNET classification type 2B

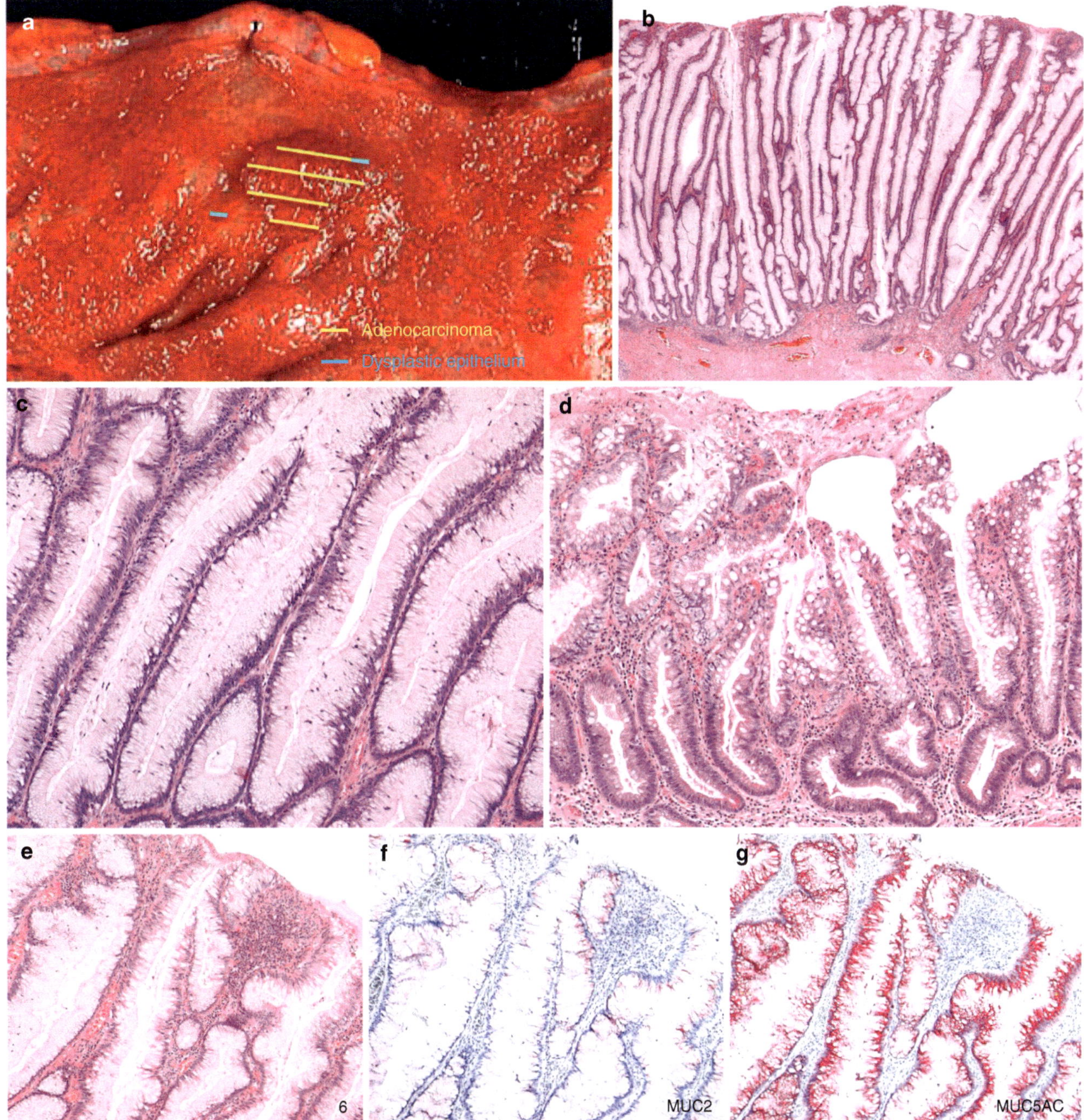

Fig. 8 Pathological image. (**a**) This is one of the multiple lesions. The resected specimen shows a 25 × 25 mm raised lesion the same color as the surrounding mucosa. Adenocarcinoma was shown in yellow line and dysplastic epithelium was shown in blue line. (**b**, **c**, and **e**) Histopathologically, the tumor ducts are uniformly mildly cellular and structurally atypical but show excessive intracellular mucus production, i.e., excessive differentiation. (**d**) A dysplastic epithelium was also seen in the surrounding area. (**f** and **g**) Immunohistochemistry, the tumor cells were predominantly positive for MUC5AC (**g**) rather than MUC2 (**f**), indicating a mixed gastric and intestinal mucin phenotype with a predominance of gastric mucin phenotype. Overall, it was diagnosed as a borderline malignant lesion or a very well-differentiated adenocarcinoma

Pathological Diagnosis

- Ascending colon: Type 0-Is + IIa, 25 × 25 mm, epithelial neoplasm of borderline malignancy and/or very well-differentiated adenocarcinoma with dysplastic epithelium, pTis (M), Ly0, V0, BD1, INF a, pPM0, pDM0, pN0.

Summary of this Case

A well-defined hemispheric elevated lesion with excess mucus production was a very well-differentiated adenocarcinoma.

5 Case 5: A Case of Early-Stage Carcinoma of Flat Type with Indistinct Borders

Takashi Hisabe and Hiroshi Tanabe

50s, female (17 years of illness)

Type of disease: Extensive

Colitis clinical course: Chronic continuous type

Macroscopic type: Superficial elevated type (indistinct border)

History of Present Illness

After the diagnosis of ulcerative colitis, the patient was treated with 5-ASA.

When symptoms worsened, steroids were administered, and the patient has been hospitalized four times.

Seventeen years after the onset of the disease, the patient underwent colonoscopy for early-stage colorectal cancer of the sigmoid colon with indistinct borders (Fig. 9).

The patient underwent total colorectal resection (Fig. 10).

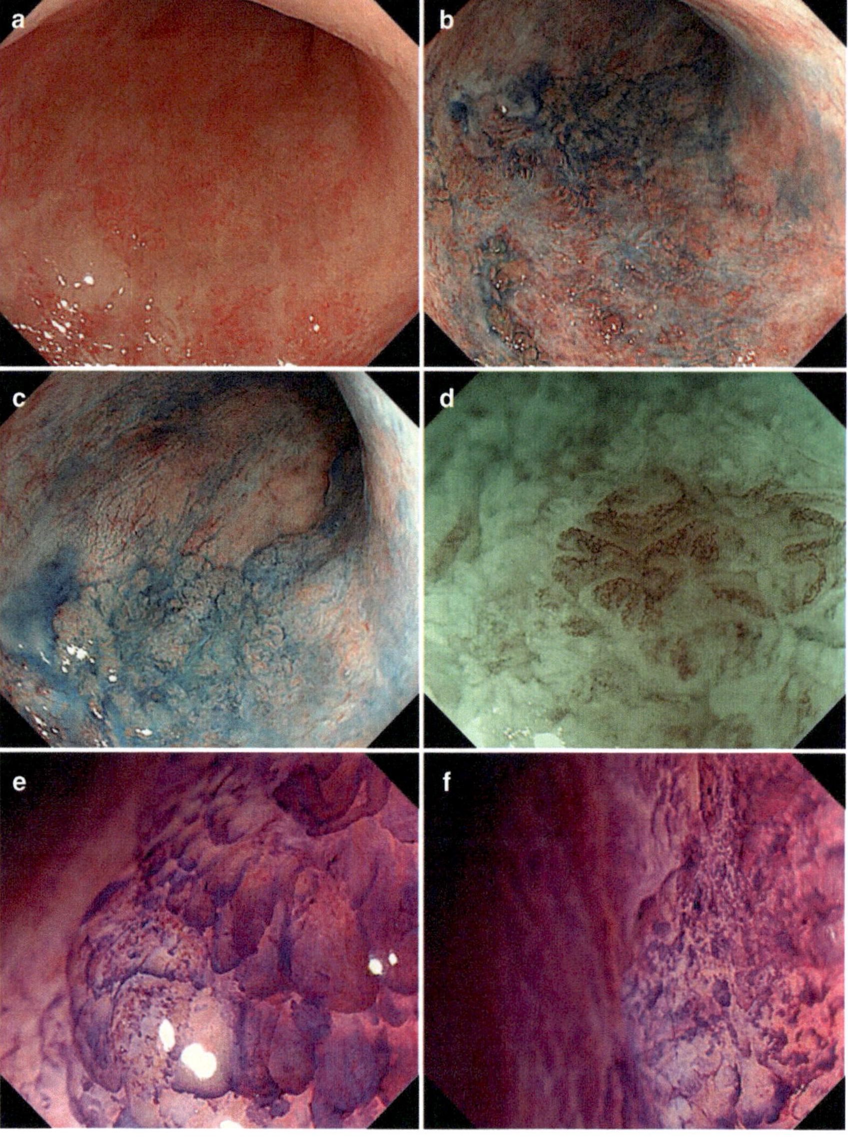

Fig. 9 Colonoscopic findings. (**a**–**c**) Conventional endoscopic observation revealed an area of mixed reddening and fading in the sigmoid colon, and chromoendoscopy revealed a low, raised lesion with indistinct borders. (**d**) NBI with ME showed extensive white opaque substance (WOS) with no visible vessel pattern, but in the observable area, the shape was uniform and the distribution and arrangement were symmetrical and regular, which was JNET classification type 2B. (**e** and **f**) The pit pattern showed irregular glandular structures in part of the type IV pit pattern, indicating V_I-low irregularity

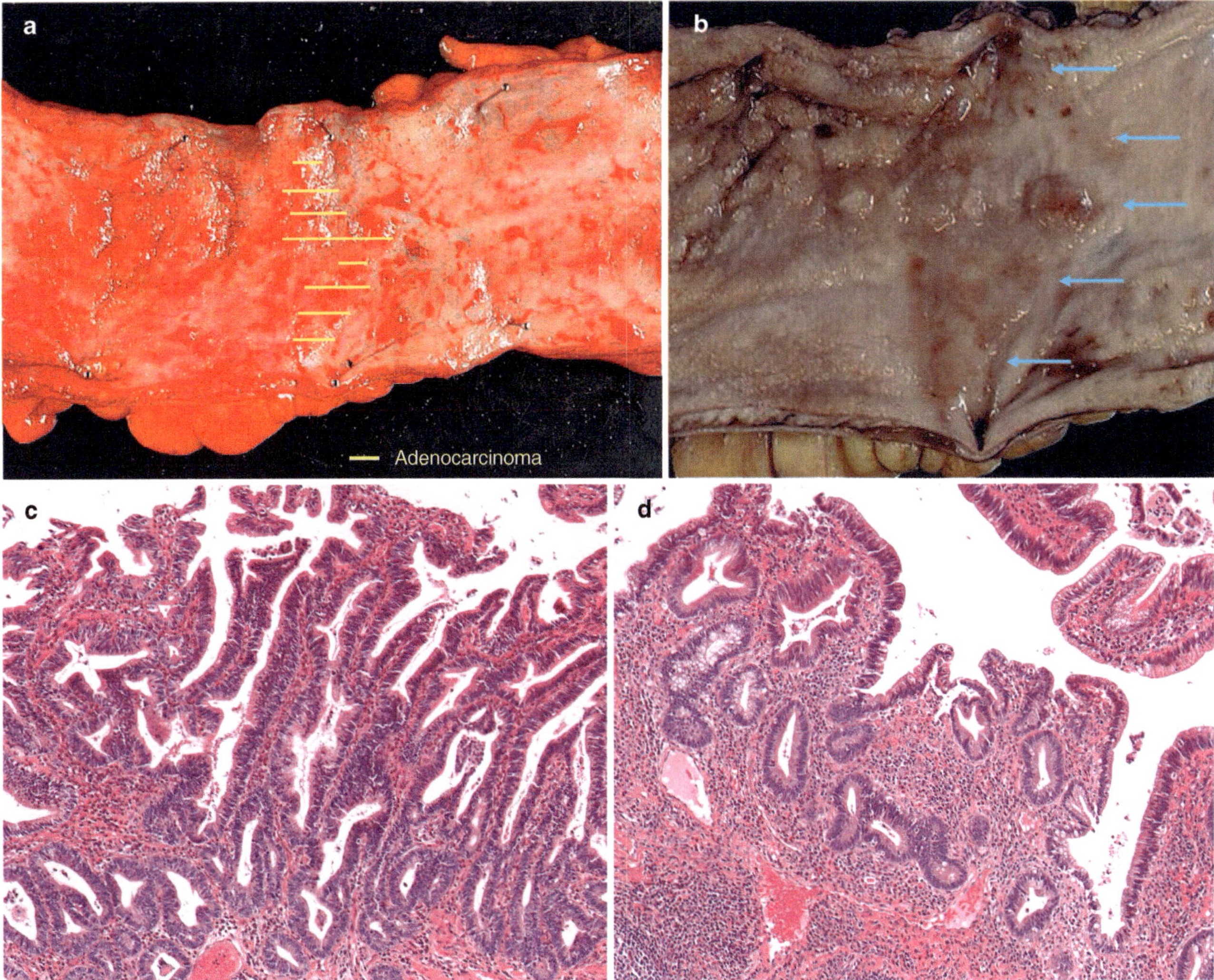

Fig. 10 Pathological image. (**a**) It is one of the multiple lesions. Adenocarcinoma was shown in yellow line. (**b**) The resected specimen shows a slightly elevated lesion, and a rough mucosa extends from the sigmoid colon to the rectum on the anal side of the lesion (arrow). (**c**) Histologically, the lesion is an intramucosal carcinoma caused by a well-differentiated tubular adenocarcinoma. (**d**) There is an extensive dysplastic epithelium on the anorectal side, which makes the borderline diagnosis of the lesion difficult. This is a typical example of multiple early-stage cancers occurring in ulcerative colitis, but it is very difficult to locate and delineate the lesions by gross morphology

Pathological Diagnosis

- Sigmoid colon: Type 0-IIa, 40 × 20 mm, well-differentiated adenocarcinoma with dysplastic epithelium, pTis (M), Ly0, V0, BD1, INF a, pPM0, pDM0, pN0.
- Stage 0: pTis, pN0, M0, P0, H0, R0, Cur A.

Summary of this Case

Endoscopic diagnosis of carcinoma of the villous protuberance was possible, but on the anal side, the boundary with the surrounding mucosa was very unclear, making it difficult to differentiate between neoplasia and non-neoplasia.

6 Case 6: Early-Stage Cancer That Was Difficult to Recognize as a Tumor

Takashi Hisabe and Hiroshi Tanabe

60s, male (15 years of illness)

Type of disease: left-sided colitis

Clinical course: Relapse-remitting type

Macroscopic type: Flat type (indistinct border)

History of Present Illness

After the diagnosis of ulcerative colitis, the patient was treated with steroids and 5-ASA.

He was steroid-dependent and was treated with granulocyte removal therapy and remained in remission.

Fifteen years after the onset of the disease, he underwent colonoscopy to evaluate the activity of the disease and was diagnosed as having colorectal cancer (Fig. 11) based on a biopsy of the colon (Fig. 12).

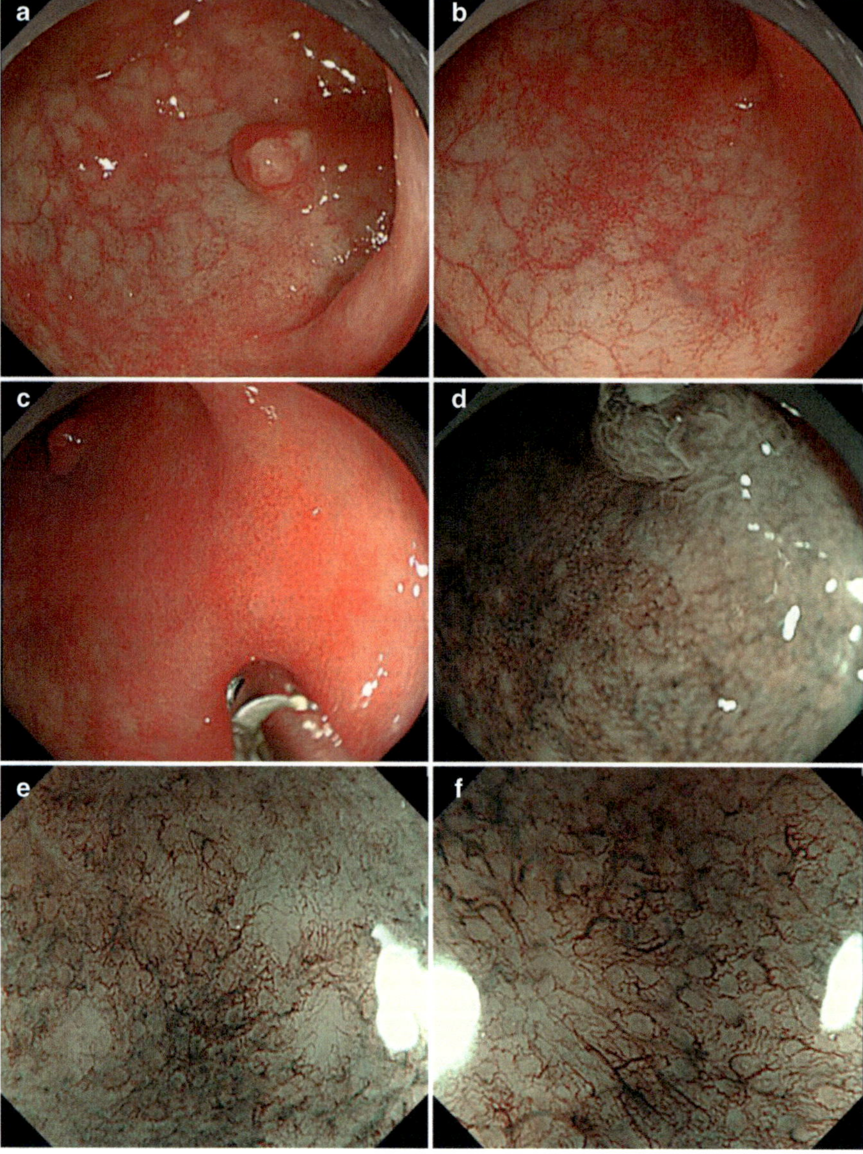

Fig. 11 Colonoscopic findings. (**a** and **b**) Conventional endoscopic observation revealed an inflammatory polyp in the sigmoid colon, with an irregular erythematous area on its anal side, and normal visible vascular images in the intervening mucosa. (**c**) Biopsy of the erythematous area on the anorectal side of the inflammatory polyp revealed a well-differentiated adenocarcinoma. (**d**–**f**) NBI with ME showed that the vessel pattern was a mixture of dendritic and tortuous microvascular architecture with honeycombed vessels surrounding a crypt opening. The surface pattern was absent. It was difficult to determine whether the lesion was inflammation or neoplasia by NBI observation

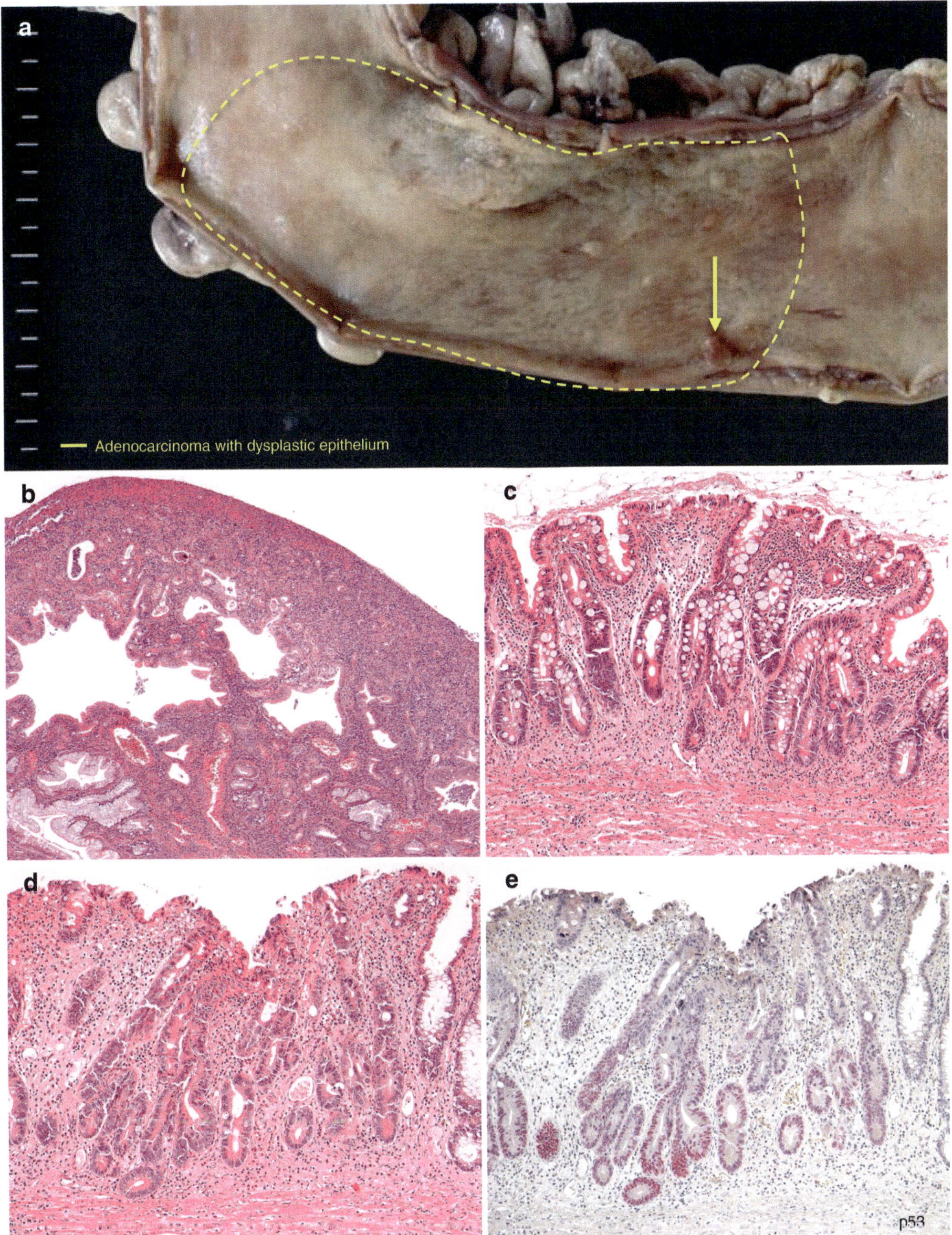

Fig. 12 Pathological image. (**a**) As in Case 5, this case has multiple lesions. In the resected specimen, the mucosa was generally atrophic and there was a small polypoid lesion in the sigmoid colon (inflammatory polyp-like elevation in the endoscopy) (yellow arrow). Flat lesion was difficult to recognize and identify grossly (yellow dot line). (**b**) Histopathologically, a small polypoid lesion within the flat lesion resembled an inflammatory polyp, but the surface showed erosions and a very well-differentiated adenocarcinoma. (**c**) Dysplastic epithelium in flat lesion. (**d**) A large area of flat lesion was very well-differentiated adenocarcinoma. (**e**) Adenocarcinomatous cells are immunohistochemically positive for p53

Pathological Diagnosis

- Sigmoid colon: Type 0-IIb + Is, 110 mm, very well to well-differentiated adenocarcinoma with dysplastic epithelium, pTis (M), Ly0, V0, BD1, INF a, pPM0, pDM0, pN0.
- Stage 0: pTis, pN0, M0, P0, H0, R0, Cur A.

Summary of this Case

The erythematous mucosa, which appeared to be inflammatory changes on endoscopy, was a mixed finding of very well-differentiated adenocarcinoma and dysplasia.

7 Case 7: Early-Stage Cancer Visible with Indigo Carmine Dye Application

Takashi Hisabe and Hiroshi Tanabe

40s, male (24 years of illness)

Type of disease: Extensive colitis

Clinical course: Chronic continuous type

Macroscopic type: flat type (indistinct border)

History of Present Illness

After the diagnosis of ulcerative colitis, the patient was treated with 5-ASA.

Twenty-four years after the onset of the disease, he had bloody stools and underwent colonoscopy. Multiple neoplastic lesions were found in the entire colon (Fig. 13), and a total colorectal resection was performed (Fig. 14).

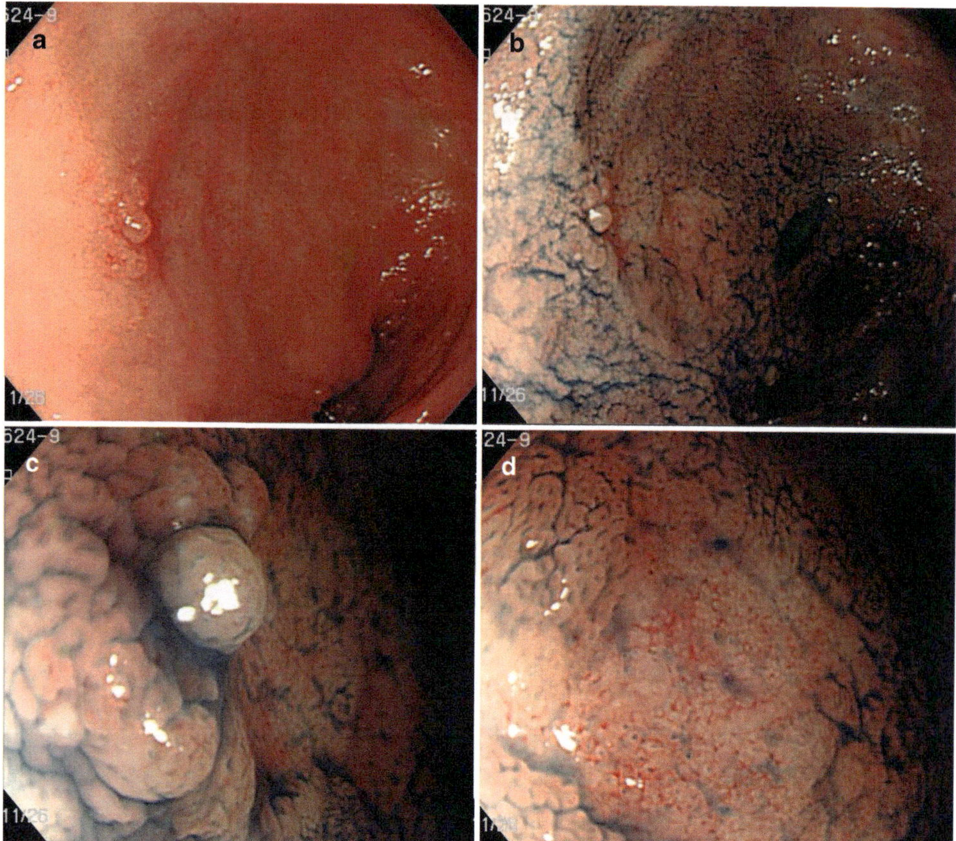

Fig. 13 Colonoscopic findings. (**a**) Conventional endoscopic examination revealed a mildly erythematous, short, raised lesion in the ascending colon. (**b**) After application of indigo carmine dye, the lesion was accompanied by a faded, flat, circular area on the anal side. (**c**) Magnification of the raised lesion revealed a gentle transition from the surrounding background mucosa with no obvious neoplastic pit. (**d**) No irregular glandular duct structure was noted in the faded area, although some type 1 pit remained

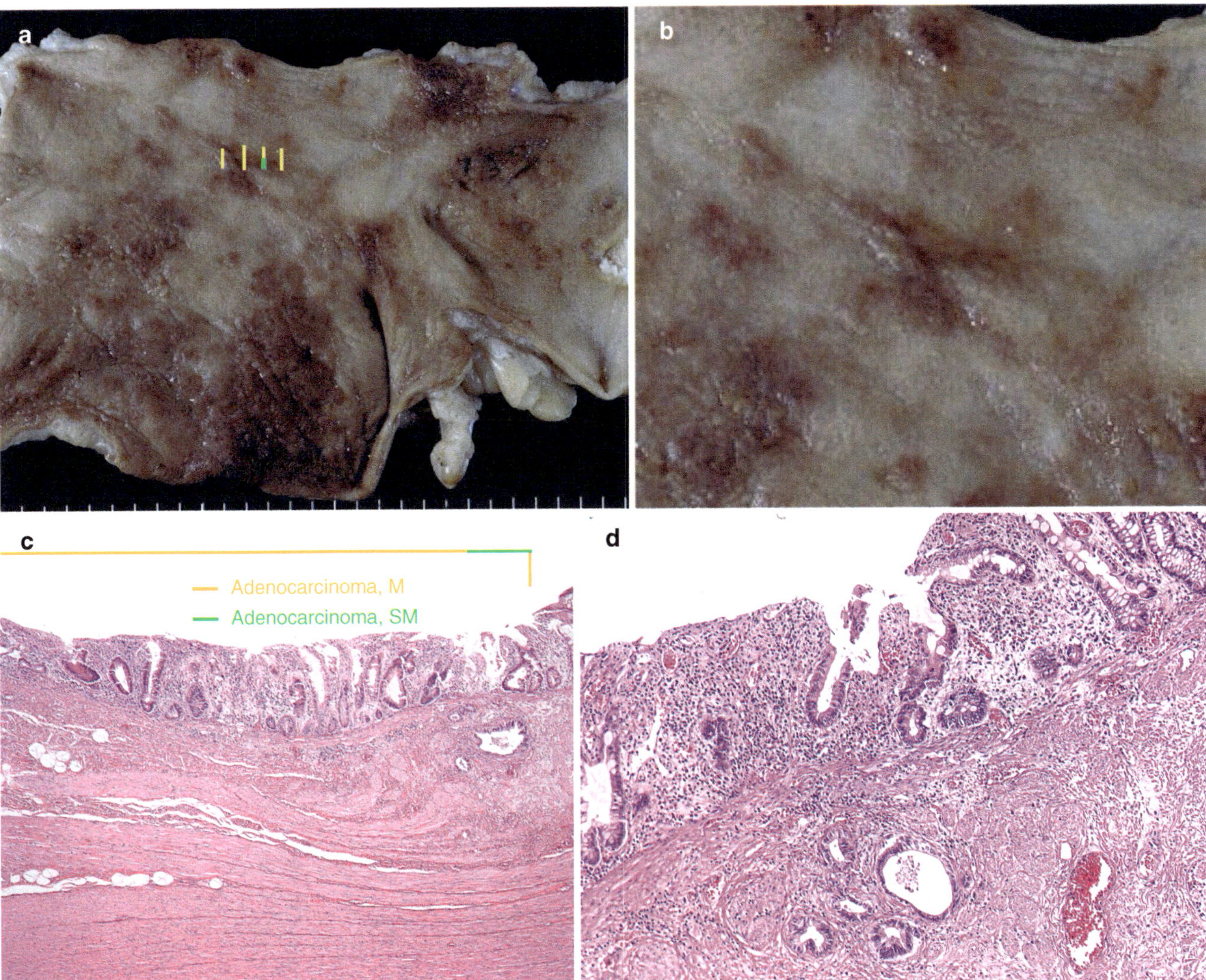

Fig. 14 Pathological image. (**a**) This is one of the multiple lesions in this patients. Adenocarcinoma was shown in yellow line and green line. (**b**) The resected specimen showed diffuse rough mucosa in the ascending colon, but the elevation seen on endoscopy was obscure, making it difficult to identify the lesion. (**c** and **d**) Histopathologically, a small well-differentiated adenocarcinoma invading the superficial portion of SM was observed. In this case, a total of six lesions including advanced cancer were identified

Pathological Diagnosis

- Ascending colon: Type 0-IIb, 15 × 10 mm, well-differentiated adenocarcinoma, pT1a (SM), Ly0, V0, BD1, INF a, pPM0, pDM0, pN0.
- Stage IIa: pT3, pN0, M0, P0, H0, R0, Cur A

Summary of this Case

The faded area with a region is a cautionary finding suspicious of UC-associated cancer, and indigo carmine spraying was useful for this lesion.

8 Case 8: Superficial Elevated Early Cancer Treated by ESD

Keisuke Kawasaki, Makoto Eizuka, Tamotsu Sugai and Takayuki Matsumoto

70-years-old female (disease duration: 33 years)

Type of disease: Total colitis

Clinical course: Relapsing-remitting type

Macroscopic type: Superficial elevated type (distinct border)

History of Present Illness

She was diagnosed as having ulcerative colitis of the total colitis type for more than 30 years and was treated with 5-ASA. At the age of 70, a surveillance colonoscopy revealed an elevated lesion in the rectum (Fig. 15) and barium examination confirmed no lateral rigidity (Fig. 16). ESD was performed (Fig. 17).

Based on the above, we diagnosed an intramucosal lesion consisting of a granular elevated lesion and a slightly elevated lesion extending to the oral side, and ESD was performed.

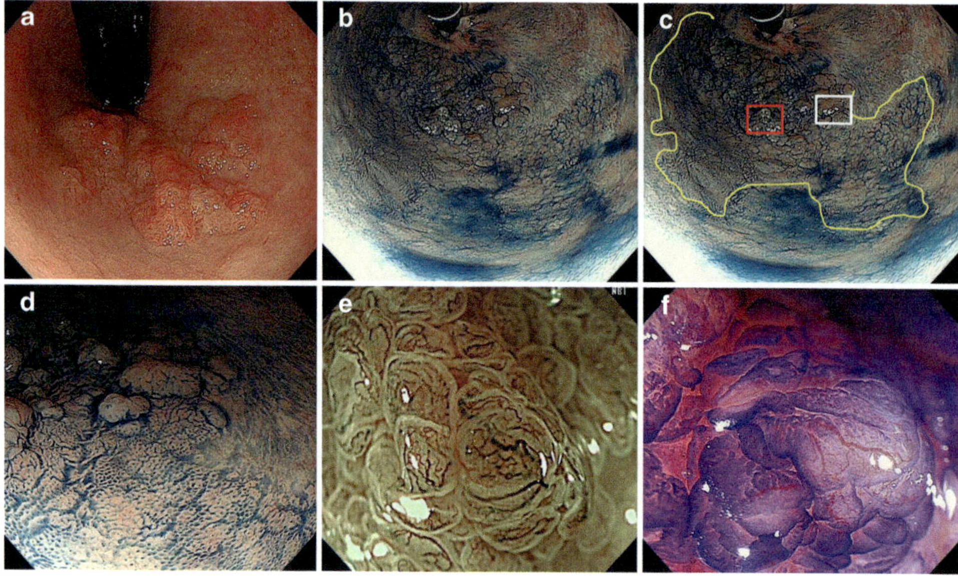

Fig. 15 Colonoscopic findings. (**a**) A granular elevated lesion consisting of erythematous areas and areas of the same color as the surrounding mucosa are seen in the lower rectum. (**b**) Chromoendoscopic findings with indigo carmine dye reveals that a fine granular mucosa extended further to the oral side of the granular ridge. The anal side is partially covered by the anal canal. (**c**) The yellow line is the oral side boundary. (**d**) Endoscopic view of the white box in (**c**). A flattened lesion slightly elevated above the surrounding mucosa, which is well-defined by dye spreading, extends further oral side of the granular elevation. (**e**) Magnifying endoscopic image with NBI of the red frame in (**c**). It was villous in shape with some enlarged vessels. (**f**) Magnifying chromoendoscopic image with the use of crystal violet solutions of the red frame in (**c**). Villous pit is seen

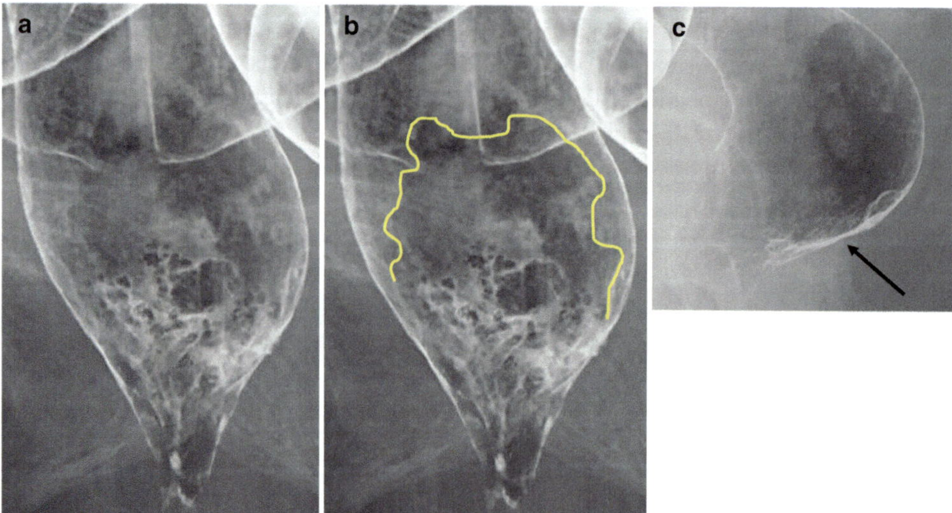

Fig. 16 Findings of barium enema examination. (**a**) An elevated lesion with a granular surface is seen on the posterior wall of the lower rectum. The granules were heterogeneous in size, and a flat lesion with a border extends to the oral of the granular elevation. (**b**) The yellow line is determined to be the oral boundary. (**c**) Wall rigidity under the profile view at the lesion is absent (arrow)

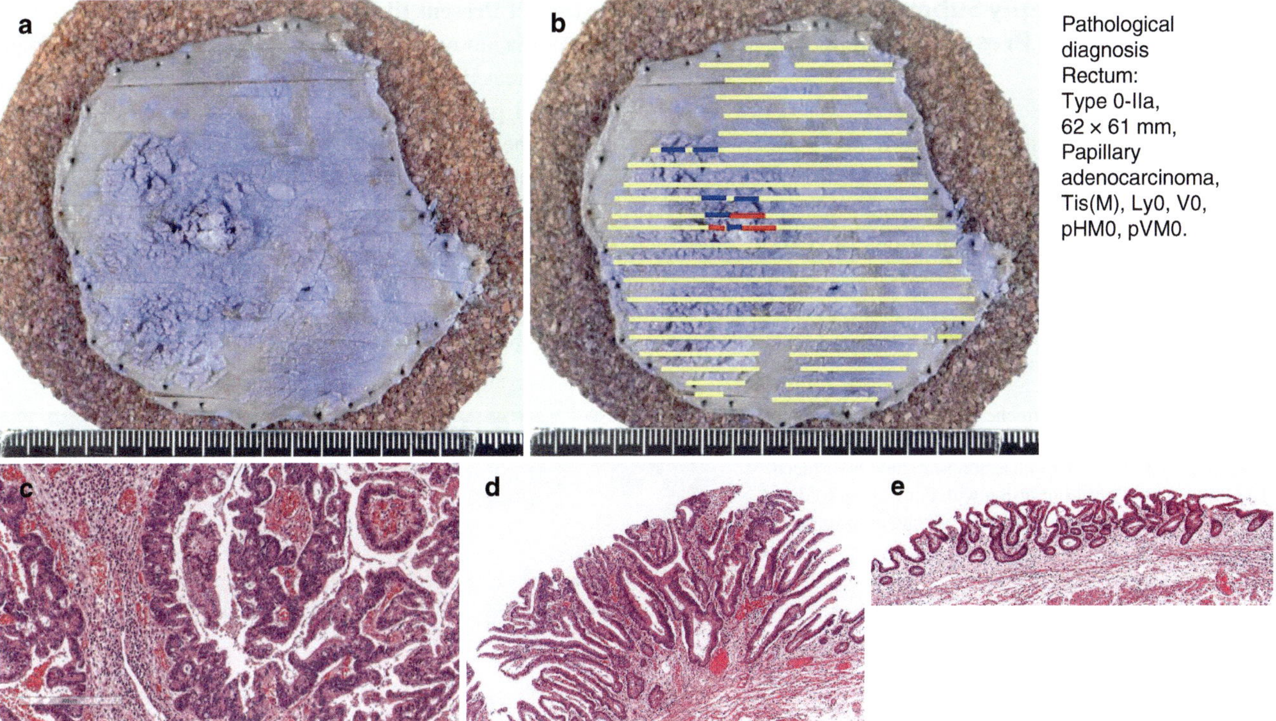

Fig. 17 Pathological image. (**a**) Resected specimen by ESD. (**b**) Mapping tumor size: 62 × 61 mm. Yellow line is low-grade dysplasia (LGD), blue line is high-grade dysplasia (HGD), and red line is papillary adenocarcinoma. (**c**) Histopathological image of the red area in (**b**). Both cellular and nuclear atypia are strong, and the morphology suggests papillary adenocarcinoma. The tumor is localized in the mucosa. (**d**) Histopathological image of the blue area in (**b**). The tubular villous structure and structural atypia are more prominent. Although both cellular atypia and structural atypia can not be diagnosed as cancer, it seems to be HGD. (**e**) Histopathology of the yellow area in (**b**). P53 is diffusely and weakly positive in carcinoma, HGD, and LGD

Pathological Diagnosis

- Rectum: Type 0-IIa, 62 × 61 mm, Papillary adenocarcinoma, Tis (M), Ly0, V0, pHM0, pVM0.

Summary of this Case

The lesion was a nodular granular lesion with microgranular mucosa extending further to the oral side, and chromoendoscopy with indigo carmine dye was useful for range diagnosis. The SCENIC consensus statement recommended endoscopic resection and post resection endoscopic surveillance for UC-associated tumors that can be resected endoscopically, although total colorectal resection has traditionally been performed for UC-associated tumors. In this case, ESD was performed because surgical resection would have resulted in an artificial anus due to the tumor's involvement in the anal canal, the patient's advanced age, and the patient's wish. Five years have passed since ESD, and the patient was currently recurrence-free.

9 Case 9: Deeply Submucosal Invasive Carcinoma Preserved Surface Structure

Keisuke Kawasaki, Makoto Eizuka, Tamotsu Sugai and Takayuki Matsumoto

40-years-old, male (disease duration: 24 years)

Type of disease: Left-sided colitis
Clinical course: Relapsing-remitting type
Macroscopic type: Sessile type (distinct border)

History of Present Illness

He was diagnosed with ulcerative colitis with left-sided colitis and was treated with 5-ASA. For the past 1 year, bloody stool, abdominal pain, and 7 kg weight loss were observed, and a tumor in the sigmoid colon was detected by radiography (Fig. 18) and colonoscopy (Fig. 19). He underwent subtotal colectomy with ileal pouch-anal canal anastomosis (IACA) (Fig. 20).

Although the superficial structure was preserved, it was considered to be a deep submucosal invasive carcinoma due to the presence of folds and lateral deformities on radiography. Therefore, surgical resection was performed

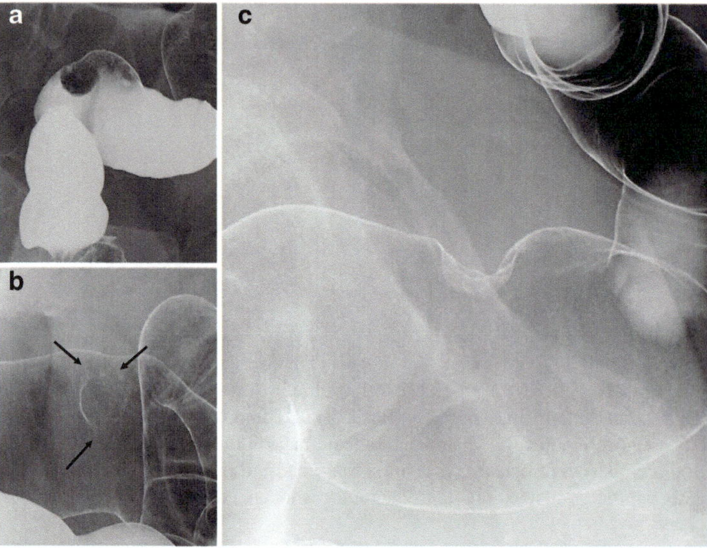

Fig. 18 Findings of barium enema examination. (**a**) Barium-filled image shows a protruding lesion in the distal sigmoid colon. (**b**) The lesion is a smooth-surfaced, 15 mm in size, protruding lesion with converging folds (arrows). (**c**) Lateral view shows an arcuate deformity

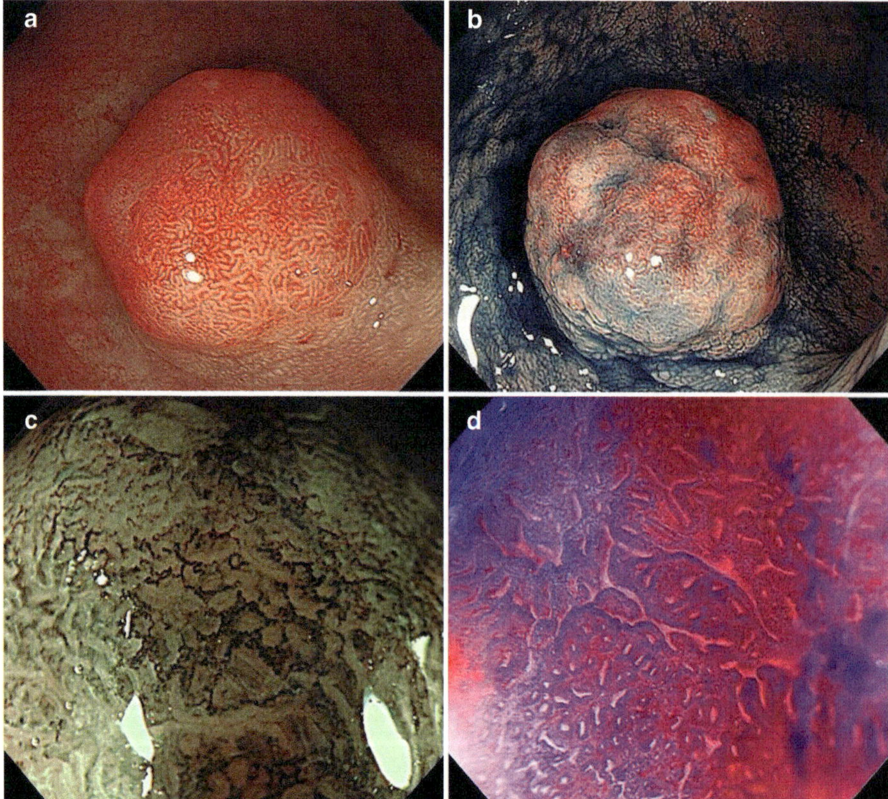

Fig. 19 Colonoscopic findings. (**a**) An erythematous protruding lesion is seen in the sigmoid colon. (**b**) In chromoendoscopic findings with indigo carmine dye, superficial structures of the lesion are preserved, and there are no dysplasias in surrounding area of the tumor. (**c**) Magnifying endoscopic image with NBI of the central part of the lesion. Both structures and vessels are clearly depicted, but there are minor vascular distortion and structural irregularities. (**d**) Magnifying chromoendoscopic image with the use of crystal violet solutions of the central part of the lesion. Tubular or dendritic pit is seen

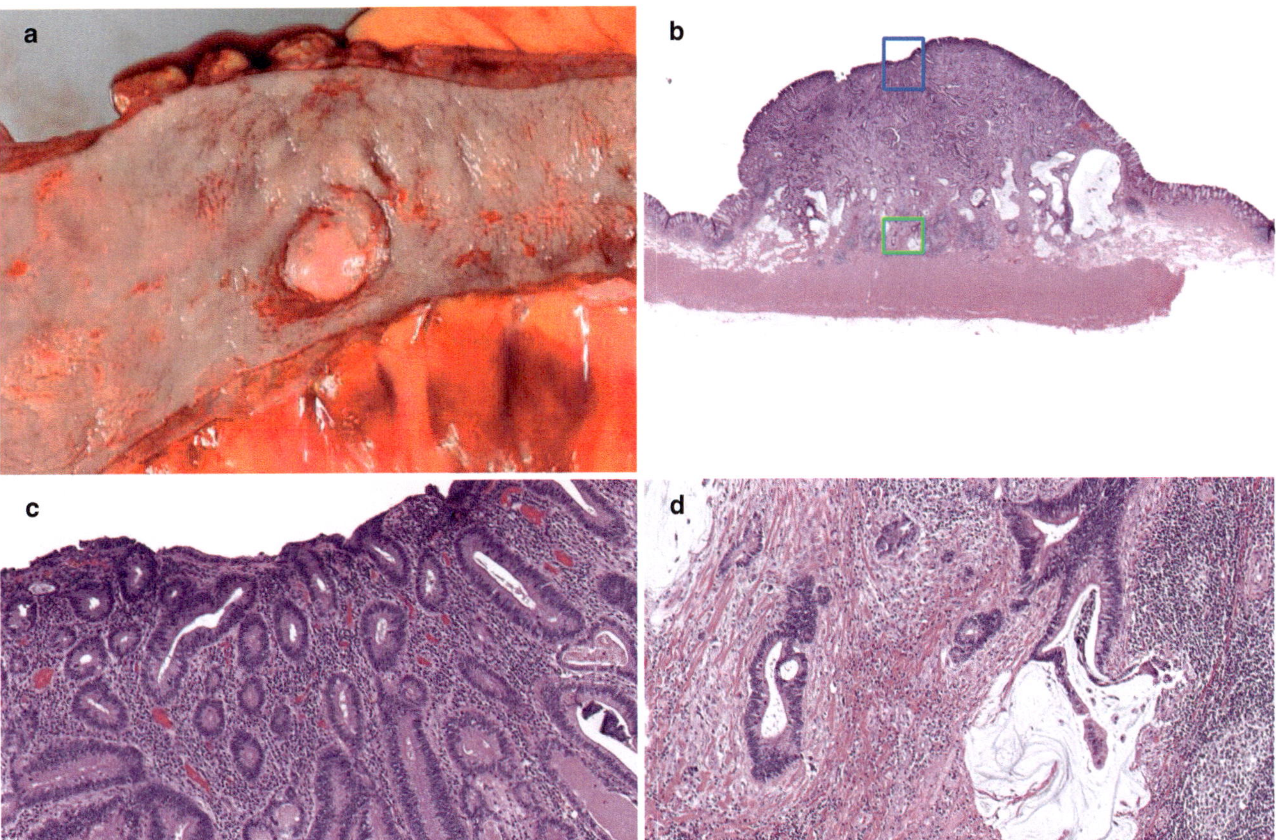

Fig. 20 Pathological image. (**a**) Resection specimen shows a protruding lesion in the sigmoid colon. (**b**) Resected specimen of loupe image. There is no dysplasia in the surrounding mucosa, and the tumor cells have infiltrated just above the muscle layer. The muscularis mucosa is torn and infiltrates up to SM 6000 μm. (**c**) Enlarged image of the blue frame in (**b**). The tumor is predominantly well-differentiated adenocarcinoma with some moderately differentiated adenocarcinoma. The superficial layers of the tumor are relatively well preserved. (**d**) Enlarged image of green frame in (**b**). Mucus production was seen in the advanced part of the tumor. P53 is negative

Pathological Diagnosis

- Sigmoid colon: Type 0-Is, 15 × 13 mm, well to moderately differentiated adenocarcinoma, pT1b (SM 6000 μm), Ly0, V0, pHM0, pVM0, pN1a.
- Stage IIIa: pT1 b, pN1a, M0, P0, H0, R0.

Summary of this Case

The tumor was located in the affected area of ulcerative colitis, and there was no dysplasia in the surrounding area. P53 was negative, and DNA methylation analysis was not performed. In this case, we considered UC-associated tumor because of the long disease duration of UC, onset of cancer at a young age, and mucus production in the advanced part of the body, but we could not determine it.

Advanced Cancers: 12 Cases with Various Features

Takashi Hisabe, Hiroshi Tanabe, Keisuke Kawasaki, Makoto Eizuka, Tamotsu Sugai, and Takayuki Matsumoto

T. Hisabe (✉)
Department of Gastroenterology, Fukuoka University Chikushi Hospital, Chikushino, Japan
e-mail: hisabe@cis.fukuoka-u.ac.jp

H. Tanabe
Department of Pathology, Fukuoka University Chikushi Hospital, Chikushino, Japan

K. Kawasaki
Department of Gastroenterology, Iwate Medical University, Iwate, Japan

Department of Medicine and Clinical Science, Graduate School of Medical Sciences, Kyushu University, Fukuoka, Japan

M. Eizuka
Department of Gastroenterology, Iwate Medical University, Iwate, Japan

Department of Molecular Diagnostic Pathology, Iwate Medical University, Iwate, Japan

T. Sugai
Department of Molecular Diagnostic Pathology, Iwate Medical University, Iwate, Japan

T. Matsumoto
Department of Gastroenterology, Iwate Medical University, Iwate, Japan

T. Matsui et al. (eds.), *Atlas of Inflammatory Bowel Disease-Associated Intestinal Cancer*,
https://doi.org/10.1007/978-981-19-3413-1_7

1 Case 10: Advanced Cancer with Difficulty in Preoperative Diagnosis of Depth of Invasion

Takashi Hisabe and Hiroshi Tanabe

70s, male (20 years of illness)

Type of disease: Extensive colitis

Clinical course: Relapse-remitting type

Macroscopic type: Sessile type (distinct border)

History of Present Illness

He was diagnosed as ulcerative colitis with left-sided colitis and was treated with steroids.

Six years after the onset of the disease, it progressed to the extensive colitis type and he had been admitted to the hospital repeatedly since then.

Twenty years after the onset of the disease, he underwent colonoscopy for surveillance and was diagnosed with colorectal cancer with multiple nodular elevated lesions in the sigmoid colon (Fig. 1) and underwent total colorectal resection (Fig. 2).

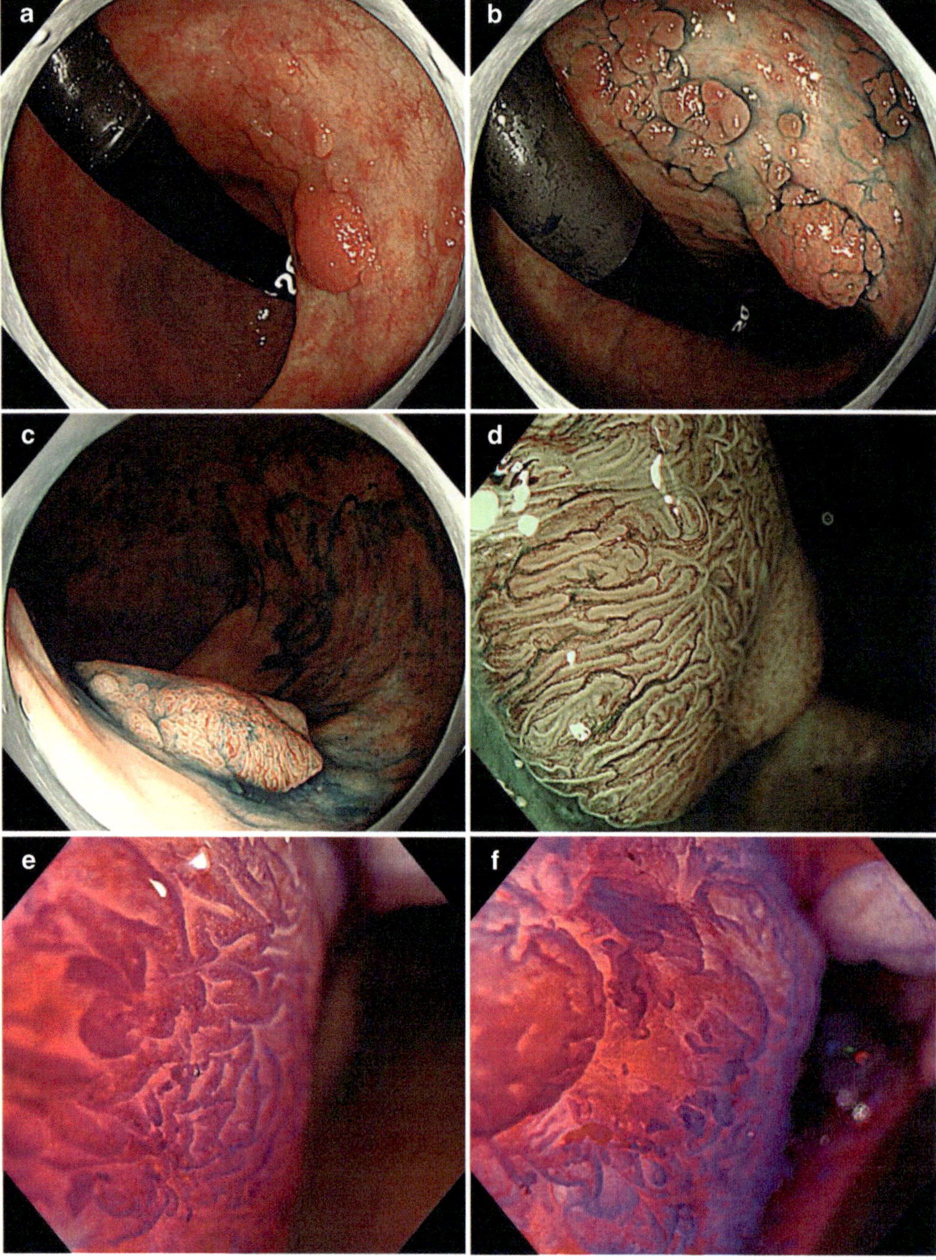

Fig. 1 Colonoscopic findings. (**a**) Conventional endoscopic examination revealed an erythematous raised lesion of 15 mm in diameter in the sigmoid colon. (**b** and **c**) Chromoendosocpy revealed a clear border of the lesion. (**d**) NBI with ME showed that the vessel pattern was uniform in shape, symmetrical in distribution and arrangement, and the surface pattern was regular with linear and arcuate epithelium at the marginal crypt epithelium, which was a JNET classification type 2A finding. (**e** and **f**) The pit pattern showed a type IV with irregular glandular duct structure in the middle, which was a type V_I-low irregularity

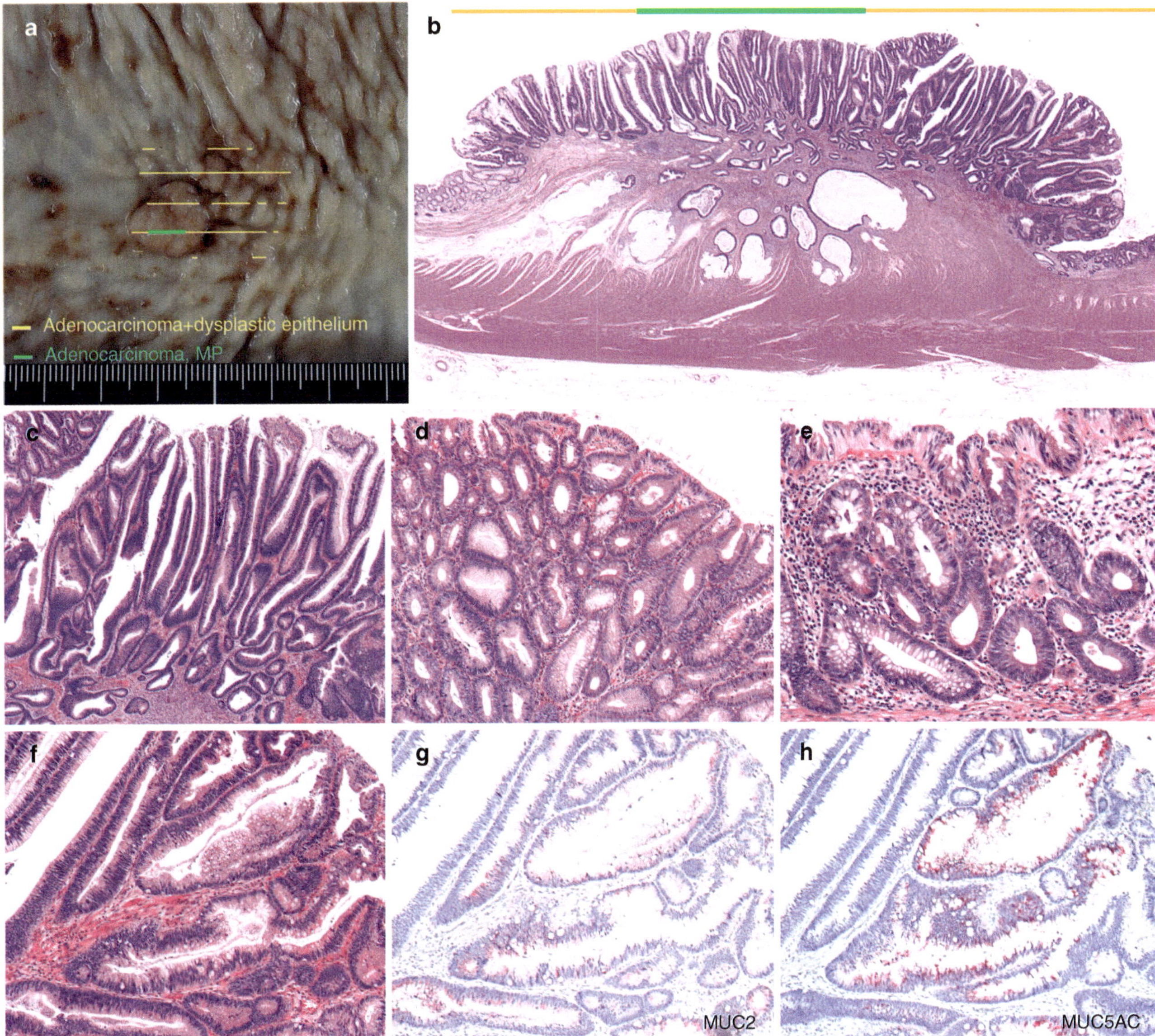

Fig. 2 Pathological image. (**a**) Yellow line shows adenocarcinoma and dysplastic epithelium, and green line shows deep invasion of the carcinoma. Grossly, it appears to be a 30 × 20 mm carcinoma with aggregate of slightly brown to same color elevations. (**b**) Lupe findings, the largest nodular elevation was an advanced carcinoma invading down into the superficial portion of the muscularis propria with extracellular mucous degeneration (**a**, **b** green line). (**c** and **f**) Histopathologically, superficial tubule-villous very well to well-differentiated adenocarcinoma. (**d** and **e**) Adenomatous areas (**d**) and dysplastic epithelium (**e**). (**g** and **h**) Immunohistochemically, the mucin phenotype of the tumor are partially positive for both MUC2 (**g**) and MUC5AC (**h**), consistent with a mixed gastric and intestinal mucin phenotype of UC-associated cancer

Pathological Diagnosis

- Sigmoid colon: Type Is + IIa-like advanced, 30 × 20 mm, very well to well-differentiated adenocarcinoma with adenomatous pattern and dysplastic epithelium, pT2 (MP), Ly0, V0, BD1, INF a, Pn0, pPM0, pDM0, pN0.
- Stage I: pT2, pN0, M0, P0, H0, R0, Cur A.

Summary of this Case

Endoscopic examination showed that the surface structure was preserved, and early-stage cancer was suspected, but advanced cancer with mucin degeneration in the muscular layer made it difficult to diagnose the depth of cancer.

2 Case 11: Type 2 Advanced Cancer with Surrounding Dysplasia

Takashi Hisabe and Hiroshi Tanabe

40s, male (30 years of illness)

Type of disease: Extensive colitis

Clinical course: Relapse-remitting type

Macroscopic type: 2 type (indistinct border)

History of Present Illness

After the diagnosis of ulcerative colitis, the patient was treated with 5-ASA, but he did not visit our hospital thereafter.

Thirty years after the onset of the disease, he had bloody stools and diarrhea and underwent colonoscopy. He was diagnosed with colorectal cancer (Fig. 3) and underwent a total colorectal resection (Fig. 4).

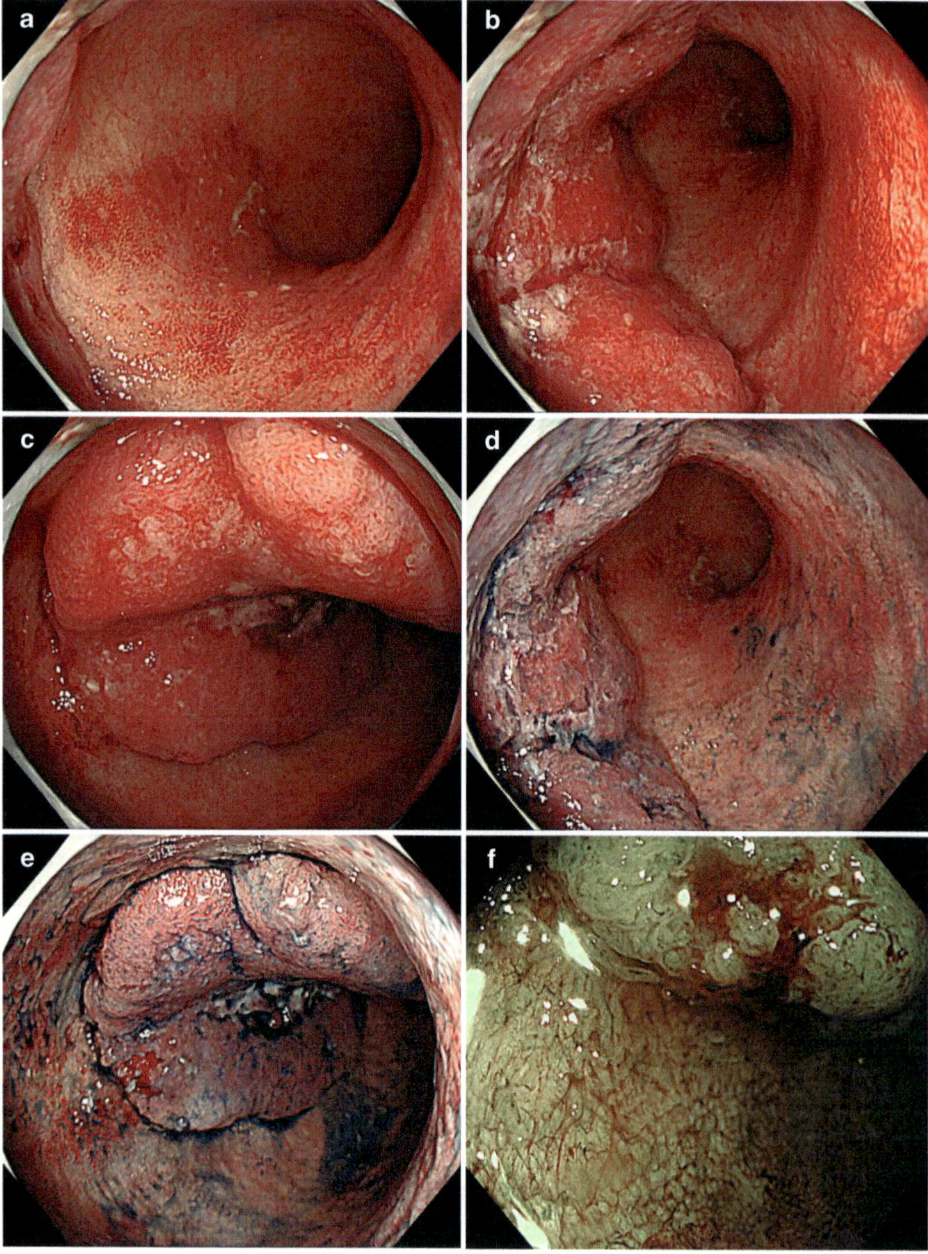

Fig. 3 Colonoscopic findings. (**a**–**c**) Conventional endoscopic examination revealed a large raised lesion in the rectum with a half circumferential occupying with an irregular ulcer in the middle. The background mucosa from the oral side of the lesion was erythematous and rough. (**d** and **e**) Chromoendoscopy revealed the boundaries of the lesions were relatively clear. (**f**) NBI with ME of the erythematous mucosa in the background showed that the vessel pattern was nonuniform in shape and irregular in distribution and arrangement, and the surface pattern was not visible, which was a JNET classification type 2B

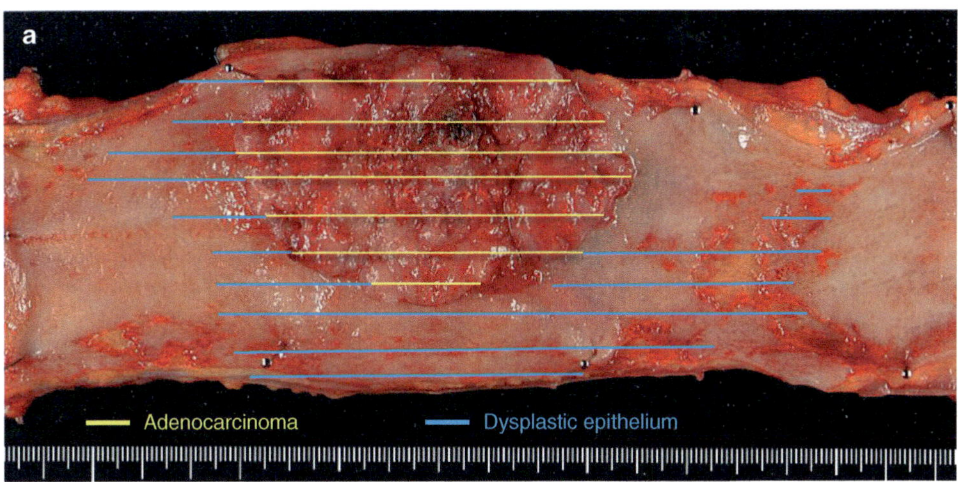

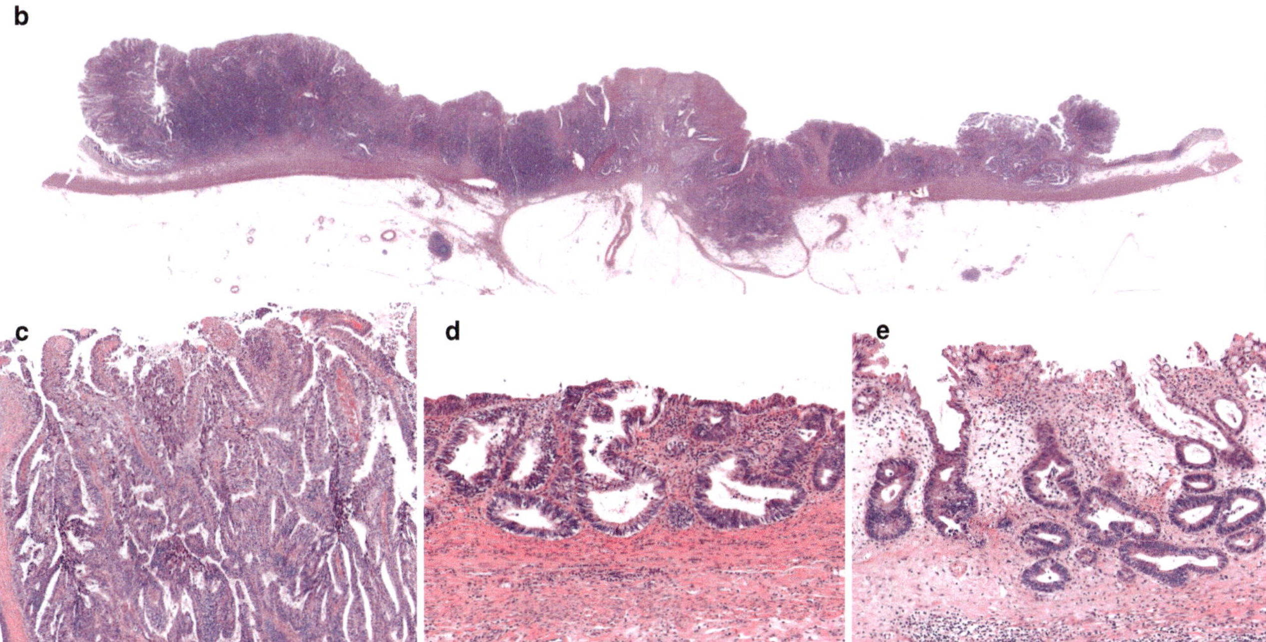

Fig. 4 Pathological image. (**a**) Grossly, the lesion resembles a sporadic type 2 advanced carcinoma (yellow line), but dysplastic epithelium was seen in the surrounding mucosa (blue line). (**b**) Lupe findings, the carcinoma was invaded whole layer of the rectum. (**c**) Histopathologically, well to moderately differentiated tubular adenocarcinoma of intestinal type. (**d** and **e**) Dysplastic epithelium was seen in the surrounding mucosa

Pathological Diagnosis

- Rectum: Type 2, 80 × 50 mm, well to moderately differentiated adenocarcinoma with dysplastic epithelium, pT3 (SS), Ly1a, V0, BD2, INF a, Pn1a, pPM0, pDM0, pN1a.
- Stage IIIa: pT3, pN1a, M0, P0, H0, R0, Cur A.

Summary of this Case

UC-associated carcinoma with dysplasia and surrounding rough mucosa, although sporadic advanced carcinoma could not be ruled out by endoscopy.

3 Case 12: Advanced Carcinoma Invading the Serosa with Difficulty in Preoperative Diagnosis of Depth

Takashi Hisabe and Hiroshi Tanabe

30s, male (13 years of illness)

Type of disease: Extensive colitis

Clinical course: Chronic continuous type

Macroscopic type: Flat type (indistinct border)

History of Present Illness

The patient was diagnosed as ulcerative colitis with left-sided colitis and was treated with 5-ASA. He continued to have symptoms and was steroid-dependent thereafter.

Eight years after the onset of the disease, he was treated with anti-TNF-α agents.

Thirteen years after the onset of the disease, he underwent colonoscopy for surveillance purposes. He was diagnosed as having colorectal cancer (Fig. 5) and underwent a total colorectal resection (Fig. 6).

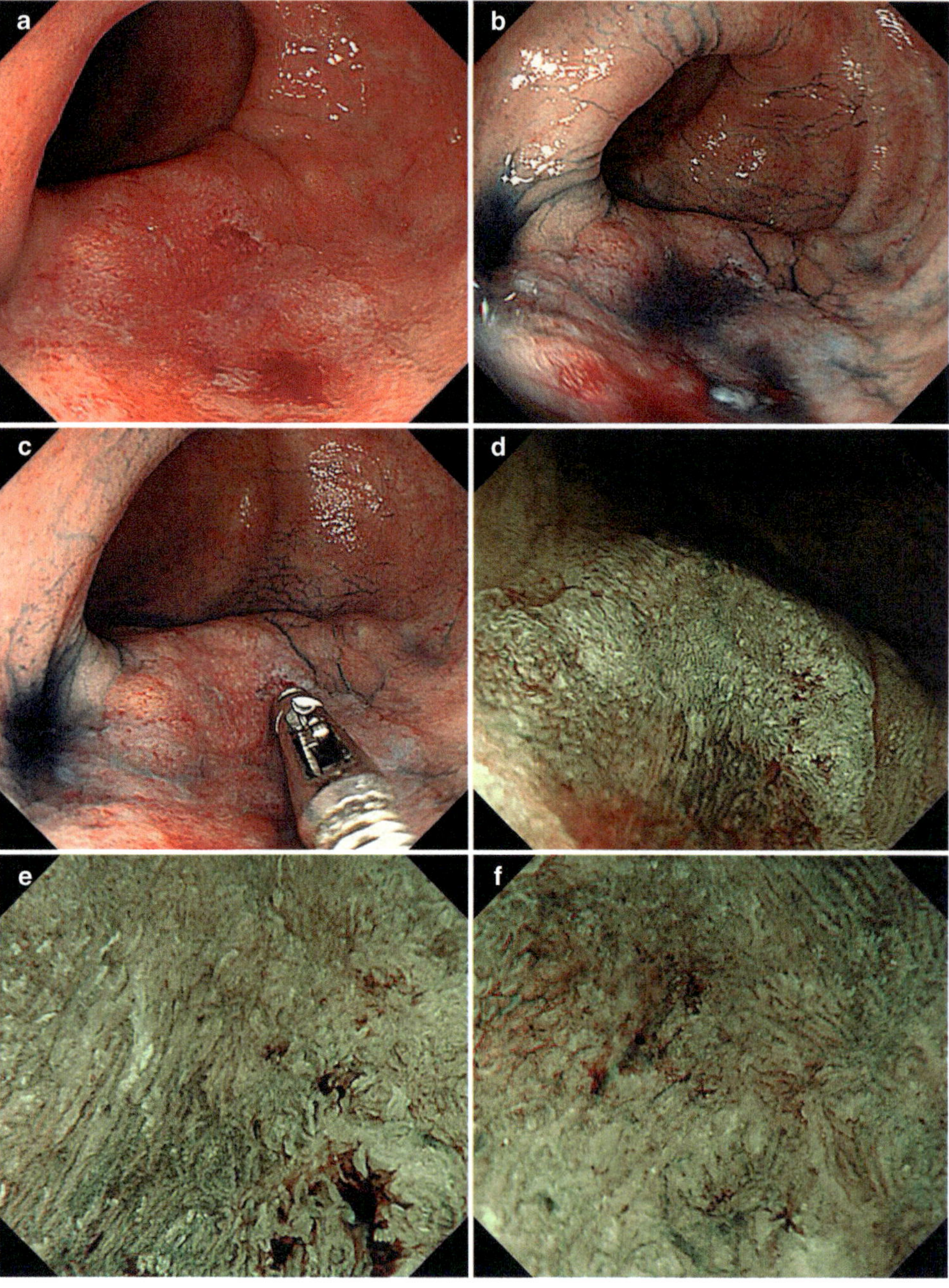

Fig. 5 Colonoscopic findings. (**a**) Conventional endoscopy revealed a flat-elevated lesion with friability in the transverse colon. (**b** and **c**) Choromoendosocy revealed a clear margin and fold convergence. (**d–f**) NBI with ME revealed a vessel pattern that was irregular, asymmetrical, and irregular in shape, size, distribution, and arrangement. The surface pattern showed irregular marginal crypt epithelium and invisible areas, which was a JNET classification type 3

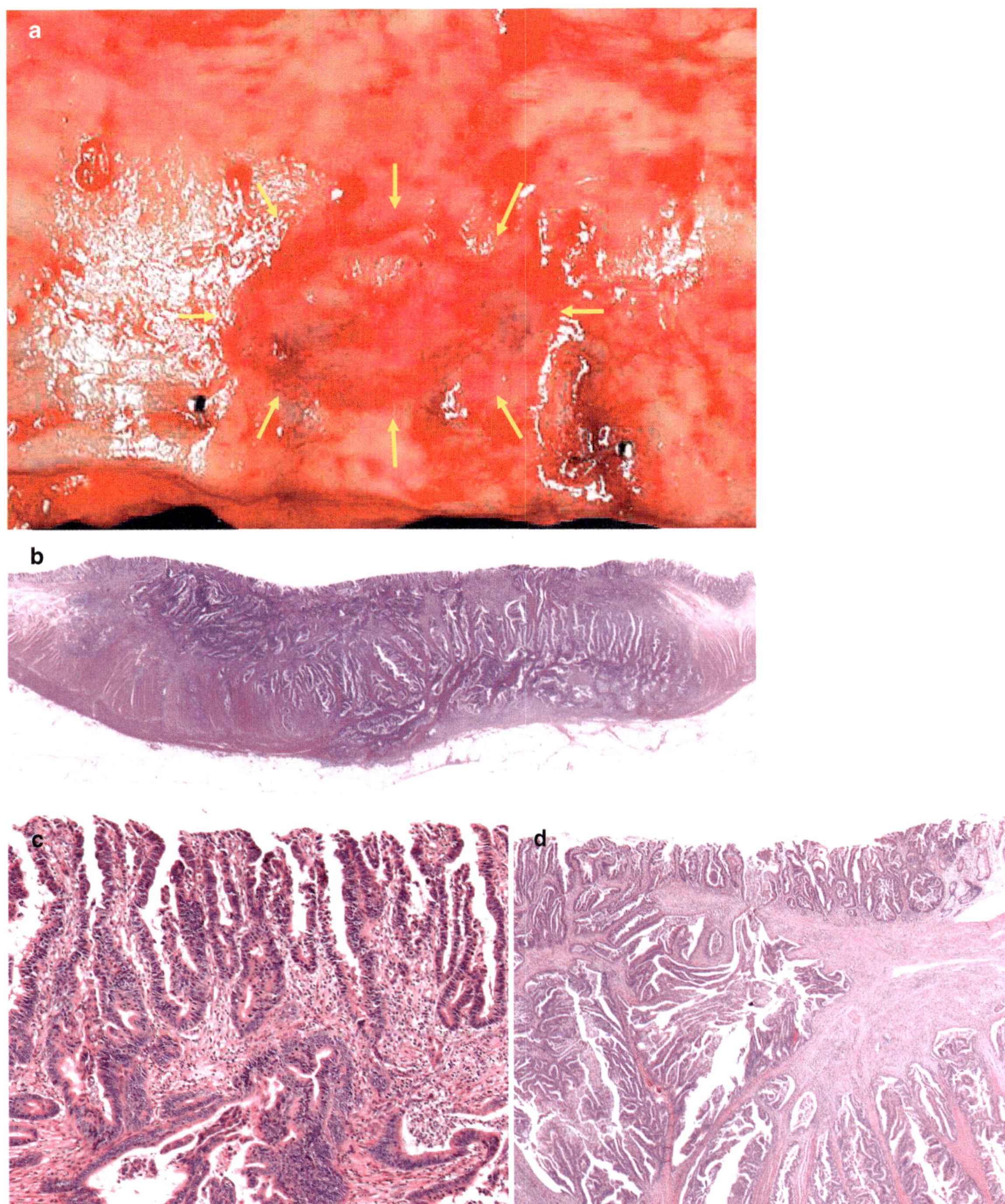

Fig. 6 Pathological image. (**a**) The lesion is one of the multiple lesions. There is an oval-shaped mild depression extending along the long axis of the transverse colon (arrows). (**b**) Lupe finding, this lesion was advanced carcinoma invading whole layer of the transverse colon. (**c** and **d**) Histophathologically, no erosions or ulcers were formed (**c**), and the mucosal lamina propria remained relatively intact except near the center of the tumor (**d**), which may have made it difficult to diagnose the depth of the tumor on gross examination

Pathological Diagnosis

- Transverse colon: Type 5, 30 × 20 mm, well to moderately differentiated adenocarcinoma, pT3 (SS), Ly1b, V0, BD2, INF b, Pn1a, pPM0, pDM0, pN1b.
- Stage IIIb: pT3, pN1b, M0, P0, H0, R0, Cur A.

Summary of this Case

Endoscopic examination revealed a flat lesion with low length, but it was difficult to diagnose the depth of the carcinoma because it had invaded the entire layer with intramucosal lesions.

4 Case 13: Advanced Cancer with Indistinct Borders

Takashi Hisabe and Hiroshi Tanabe

30s, male (13 years of illness)

Type of disease: Extensive colitis

Clinical course: Chronic continuous type

Macroscopic type: Superficial elevated type (indistinct border)

History of Present Illness

He was diagnosed as ulcerative colitis with left-sided colitis and was treated with 5-ASA. The patient continued to have symptoms and was steroid-dependent.

Eight years after the onset of the disease, the patient was treated with anti-TNF-α agents.

Thirteen years after the onset of the disease, the patient underwent colonoscopy for surveillance purposes. The patient was diagnosed as having colorectal cancer (Fig. 7) and underwent a total colorectal resection (Fig. 8).

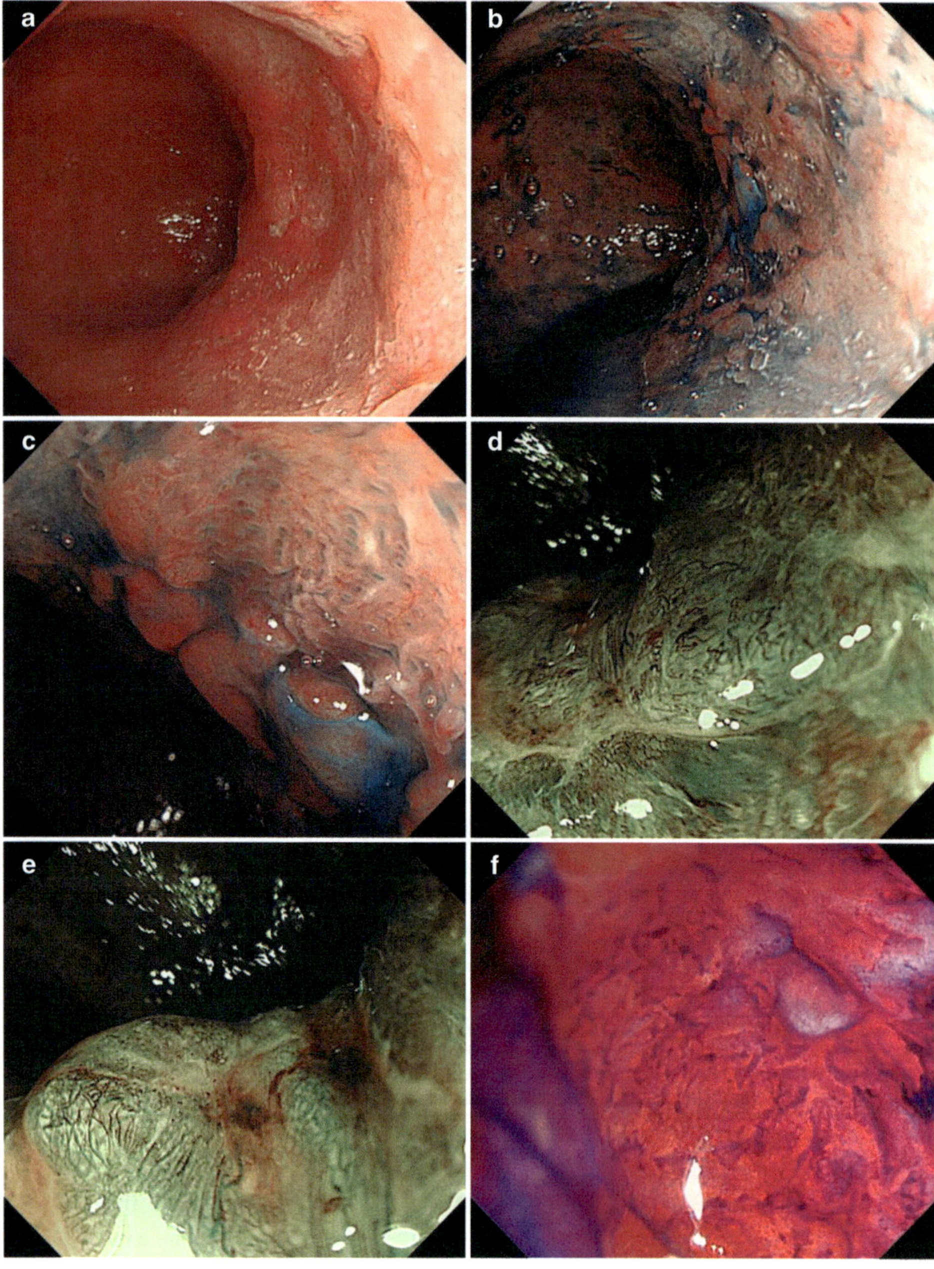

Fig. 7 Colonoscopic findings. (**a**) Conventional endoscopic examination revealed an erythematous coarse mucosa with erosions in the sigmoid colon. (**b** and **c**) Choromoendoscopy revealed a granular, superficially elevated lesion with indistinct. Weak magnification showed fine granules and velvety morphology. (**d** and **e**) NBI with ME of the central part of the lesion showed that the vessel pattern was irregular with asymmetric distribution and arrangement, and the surface pattern was not visible, which was a JNET classification type 2B finding. (**f**) The pit pattern was V_I-high irregularity to V_N

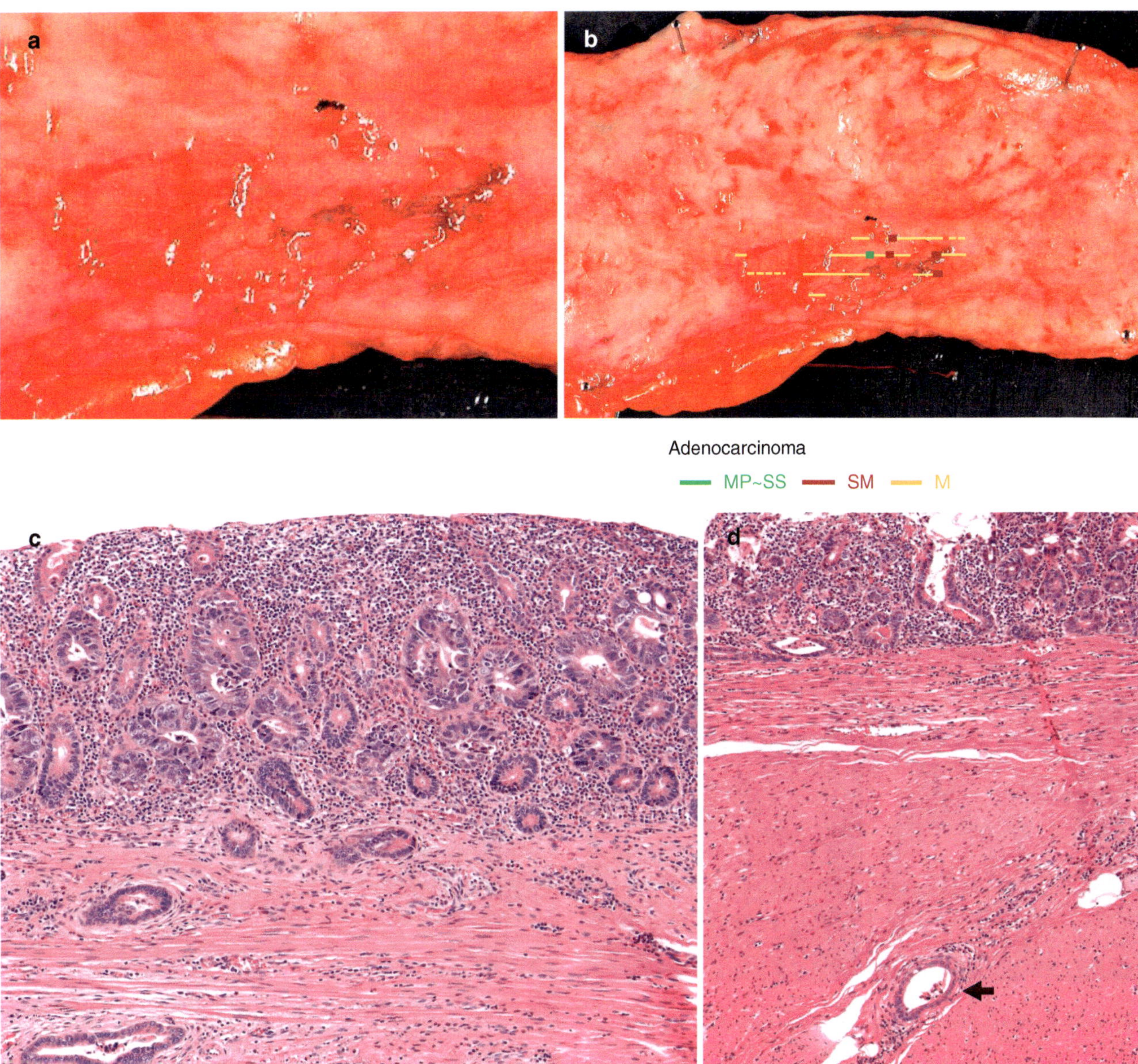

Fig. 8 Pathological image. (**a**) This is the same case as Case 10, with a very slightly elevated lesion in the sigmoid colon. (**b**) Yellow line shows intramucosal adenocarcinoma, and red and green line shows deep invasion of the carcinoma. (**c**) The histological type is well-differentiated tubular adenocarcinoma. (**d**) Most of the lesions are intramucosal, but there is some invasion into the muscularis propria (arrow)

Pathological Diagnosis

- Sigmoid colon: IIa-like advanced, 55 × 15 mm, well-differentiated adenocarcinoma, pT2 (MP), Ly1a, V0, BD1, INF a, Pn0, pPM0, pDM0.

Summary of this Case

A slightly elevated lesion with indistinct borders on endoscopy was suspected to be an early-stage cancer, but it was advanced cancer with partial invasion into the intrinsic muscle layer.

5 Case 14: Advanced Cancer Followed Up as an Inflammatory Polyp

Takashi Hisabe and Hiroshi Tanabe

50s, male (5 years of illness)

Type of disease: Extensive colitis

Clinical course: Chronic continuous type

Macroscopic type: Type 1 (distinct border)

History of Present Illness

The patient was diagnosed with ulcerative colitis and was treated with 5-ASA.

Two years after the onset of the disease, an inflammatory polyp in the hepatic flexure was noted during a colonoscopy for activity evaluation. During the follow-up, EMR was performed on a part of the lesion for diagnostic purposes, but the neoplasia could not be diagnosed.

Five years after the onset of the disease, the lesion increased and the patient was diagnosed with advanced colorectal cancer by colonoscopy (Fig. 9) and by radiography (Fig. 10) and underwent subtotal colorectal resection (Fig. 11).

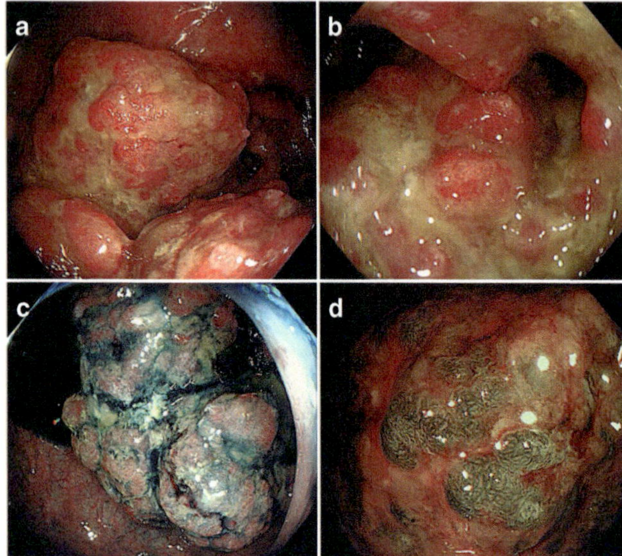

Fig. 9 Colonoscopic findings. (**a**–**c**) Conventional endoscopic observation revealed a multinodular raised lesion with erythematous surface with white exudate in the hepatic flexure. The lesion was circumferential, and the lesion itself was too hard to be scoped deeply. The surface of the lesion was smooth and there were no obvious malignant findings. (**d**) The surface pattern was regular with marginal crypt and JNET classification type 2A. The biopsy showed no malignant findings

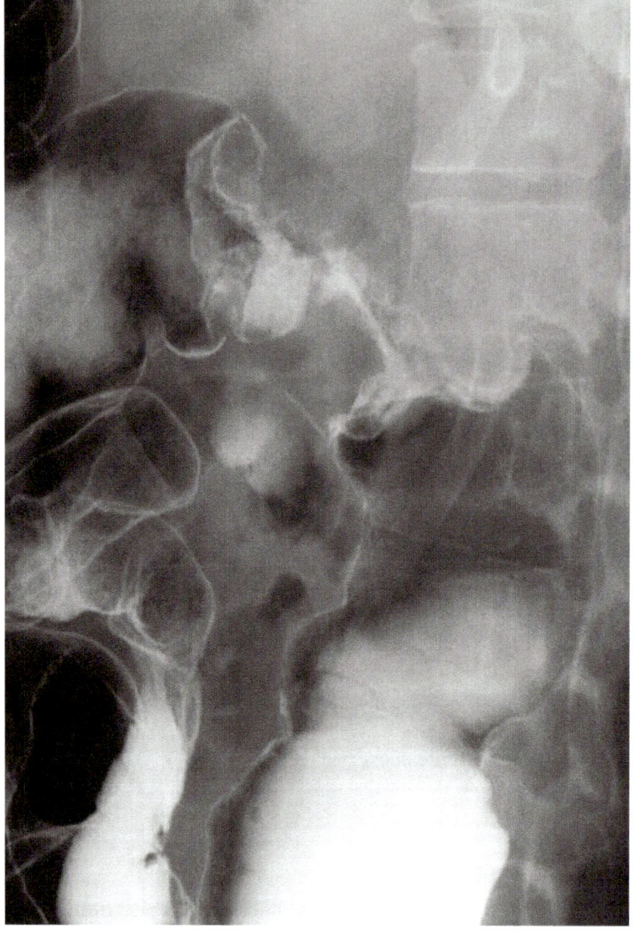

Fig. 10 Barium enema findings. Barium enema examination showed a typical apple core sign

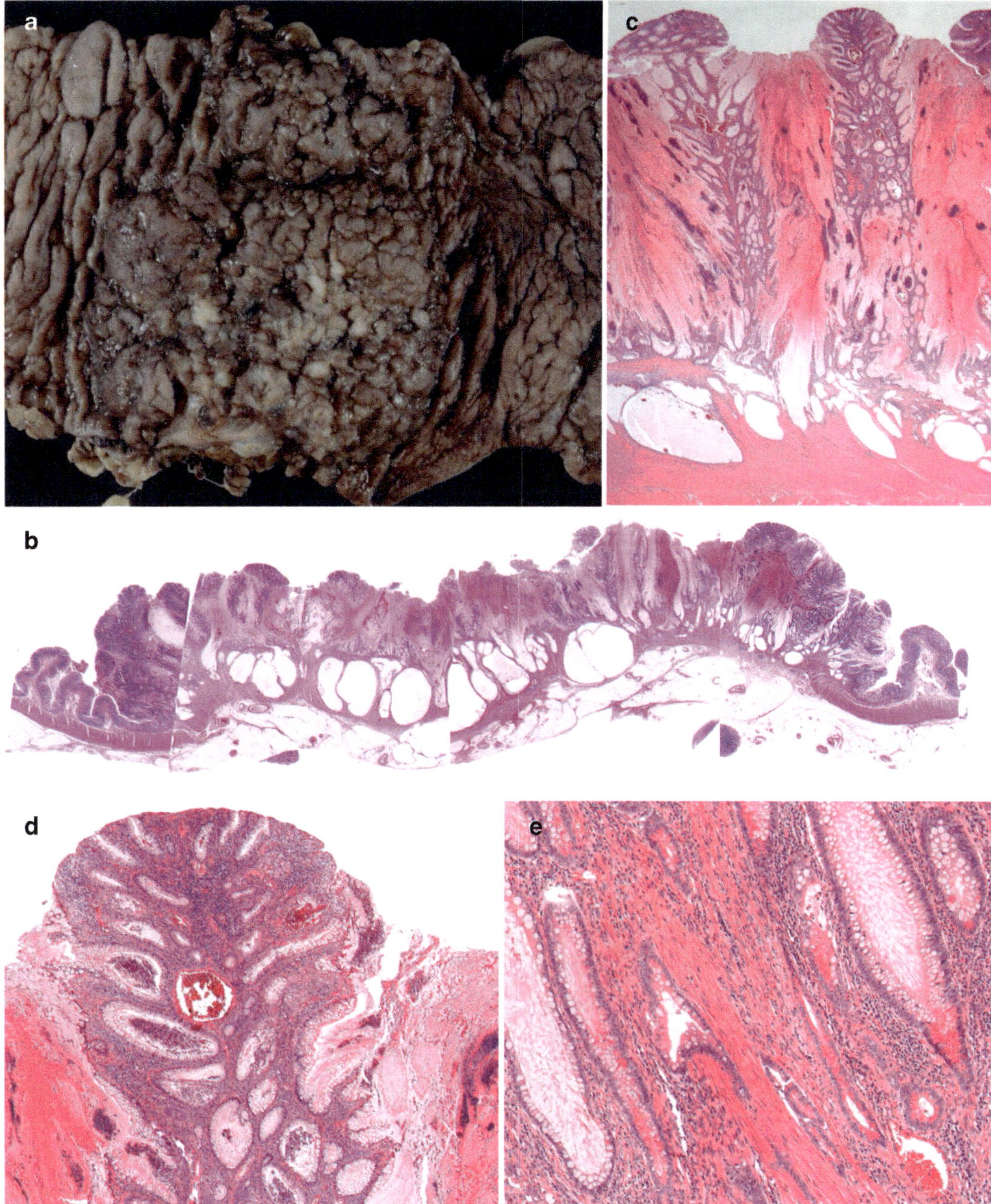

Fig. 11 Pathological image. (**a**) Grossly, a circumferential multinodular elevated lesion was found in the transverse colon. (**b**) Lupe finding, the carcinoma has invaded the subserosal layer with extracellular mucous degeneration. (**c**) The individual nodular elevations have an inflammatory polyp-like morphology, suggesting a very well-differentiated adenocarcinoma. (**d**) Tumor and nontumor epithelium are intermingled within the lesion, making it difficult to distinguish between them, and in the absence of invasion, the diagnosis of carcinoma may be difficult. (**e**) The deeper tumor ducts show excessive differentiation into Paneth cells

Pathological Diagnosis

- Transverse colon: Type 1, 80 mm, very well-differentiated adenocarcinoma with partly extracellular mucous degeneration, pT3 (SS), Ly0, V0, BD1, INF a, Pn1a, pPM0, pDM0, pN0.
- Stage IIa: pT3, pN0, M0, P0, H0, R0, Cur A.

Summary of this Case

Inflammatory polyp turned out to be cancerous, and it was very difficult to differentiate neoplasia from non-neoplasia by observation of the tumor surface layer.

6 Case 15: Advanced Cancer with Surrounding Flat Early Cancer

Takashi Hisabe and Hiroshi Tanabe

30s, female (14 years of illness)

Type of disease: left-sided colitis

Clinical course: Relapse-remitting type

Macroscopic type: Type 5 (indistinct border)

History of Present Illness

The patient was diagnosed with proctitis ulcerative colitis and was treated with 5-ASA, but he did not visit our hospital.

Twelve years after onset, the patient relapsed and 5-ASA was restarted.

Fourteen years after the onset of the disease, a colonoscopy was performed to evaluate the activity of the patient. The patient was diagnosed with advanced colorectal cancer by colonoscopy (Fig. 12) and underwent a total colorectal resection (Fig. 13).

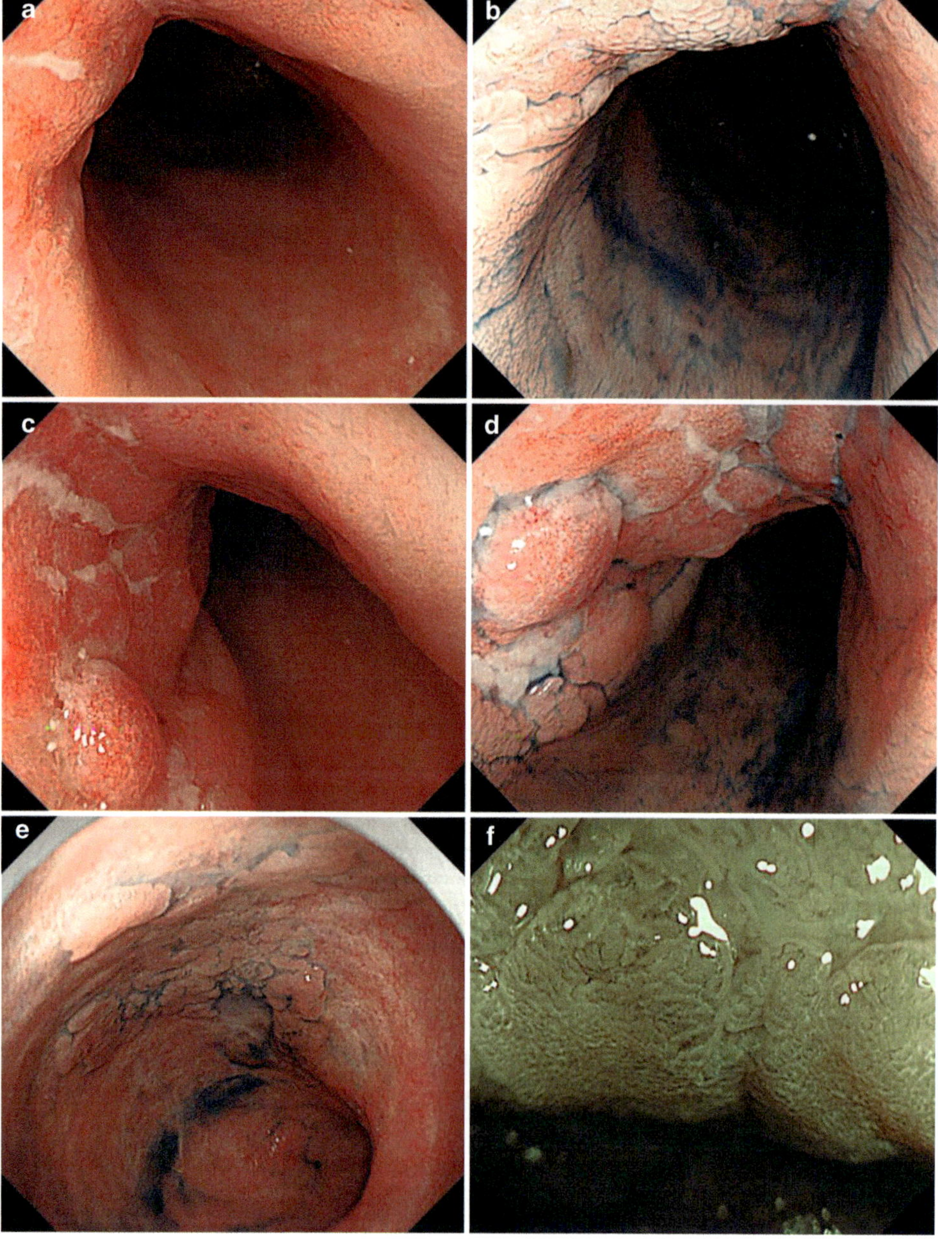

Fig. 12 Colonoscopic findings. (**a**–**d**) Conventional endoscopic observation revealed an erythematous, irregularly elevated lesion in the rectum, occupying half of the lumen, with an irregular depression. After the application of indigo carmine dye, the border of the lesion was indistinct, and extension was poor even with air pumping. (**e**) On the anal side of the lesion, there was a low, well-defined elevated lesion. (**f**) NBI with ME of the same area showed that the vessel pattern was mostly obscured by WOS, but some of the shape was uniform and the distribution and arrangement were symmetrical and regular, and the surface pattern was regular based on the uniform WOS morphology. The surface pattern was regular based on the morphology of uniform WOS, and it was judged to be a JNET classification type 2A finding

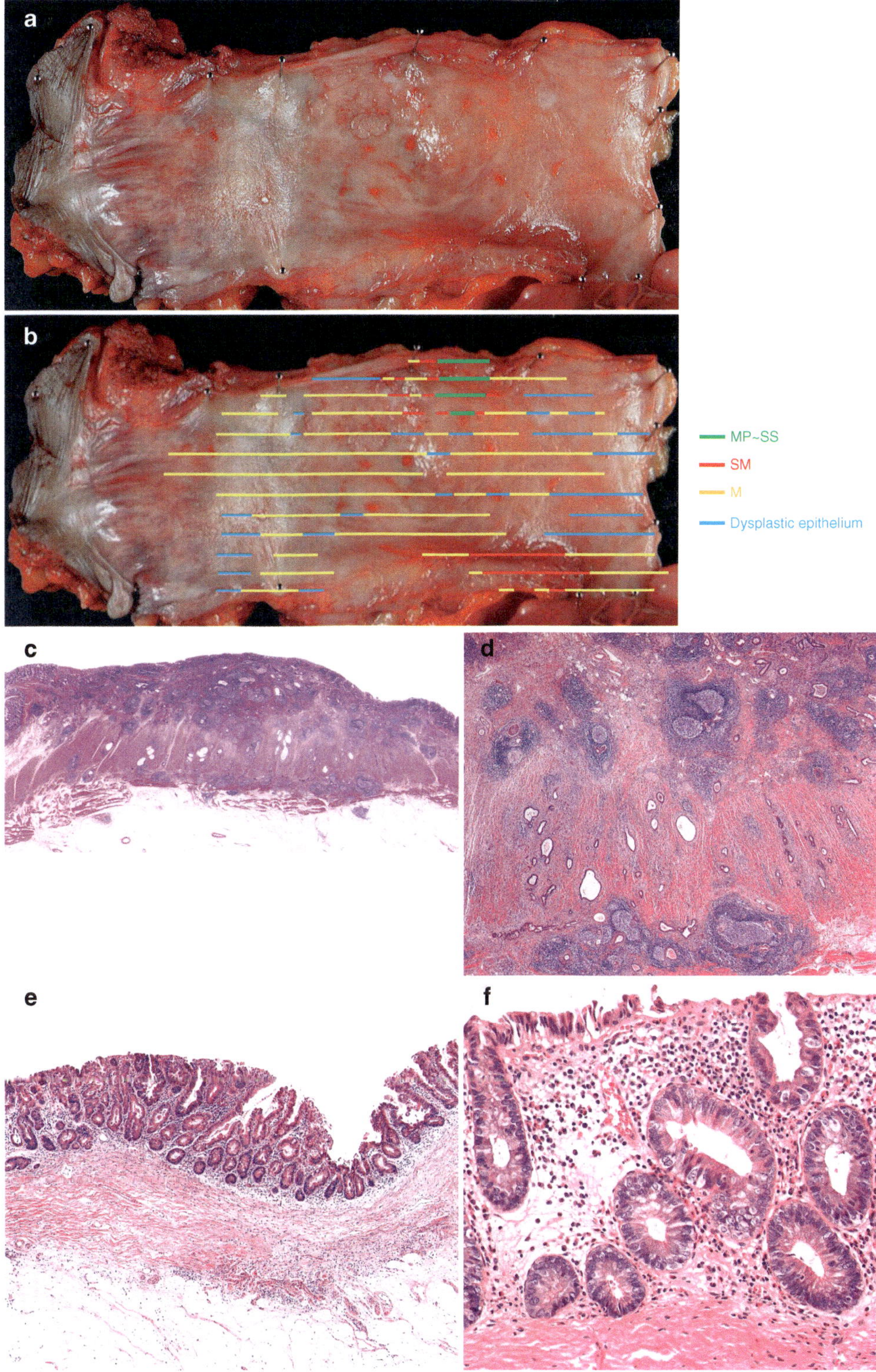

Fig. 13 Pathological image. (**a**) It is a circumferential lesion of the rectum. Grossly, there is atrophic mucosa and flattened elevation. (**b**) Schematic illustration of adenocarcinoma and dysplastic epithelium. (**c**) Lupe finding, the carcinoma has partly invaded whole layer of the rectum. (**d**) Slightly to the oral side of the flat elevation, there is an area of well-differentiated tubular adenocarcinoma invading into the subserosa, but it does not present the typical gross image of advanced cancer because the carcinoma invades like a tree root while maintaining the layered structure. (**e** and **f**) The surrounding mucosa is extensively covered with well-differentiated tubular adenocarcinoma (**e**) or dysplastic epithelium (**f**), including a flat elevation

Pathological Diagnosis

- Rectum: Type 5, 125 mm, very well to well-differentiated adenocarcinoma with dysplastic epithelium, pT3 (SS), Ly1b, V1a, BD1, INF b, Pn0, pPM0, pDM0, pN0.
- Stage IIa: pT3, pN0, M0, P0, H0, R0, Cur A.

Summary of this Case

A well-defined LST associated with the anorectal side of the main lesion, an advanced carcinoma, was also a highly differentiated adenocarcinoma.

7 Case 16: Advanced Cancer with Surrounding Flat Early Cancer

Takashi Hisabe and Hiroshi Tanabe

50s, female (25 years of illness)

Type of disease: Left-sided colitis

Clinical course: Relapse-remitting type

Macroscopic type: Type 5 (indistinct border)

History of Present Illness

The patient was diagnosed with ulcerative colitis and was treated with 5-ASA, but he did not visit our hospital thereafter.

Twenty-five years after the onset of the disease, the patient developed upper abdominal pain and diarrhea and underwent colonoscopy, which revealed multiple irregular elevated lesions in the colon. The patient was diagnosed with advanced colorectal cancer by colonoscopy (Fig. 14) and underwent a total colorectal resection (Fig. 15).

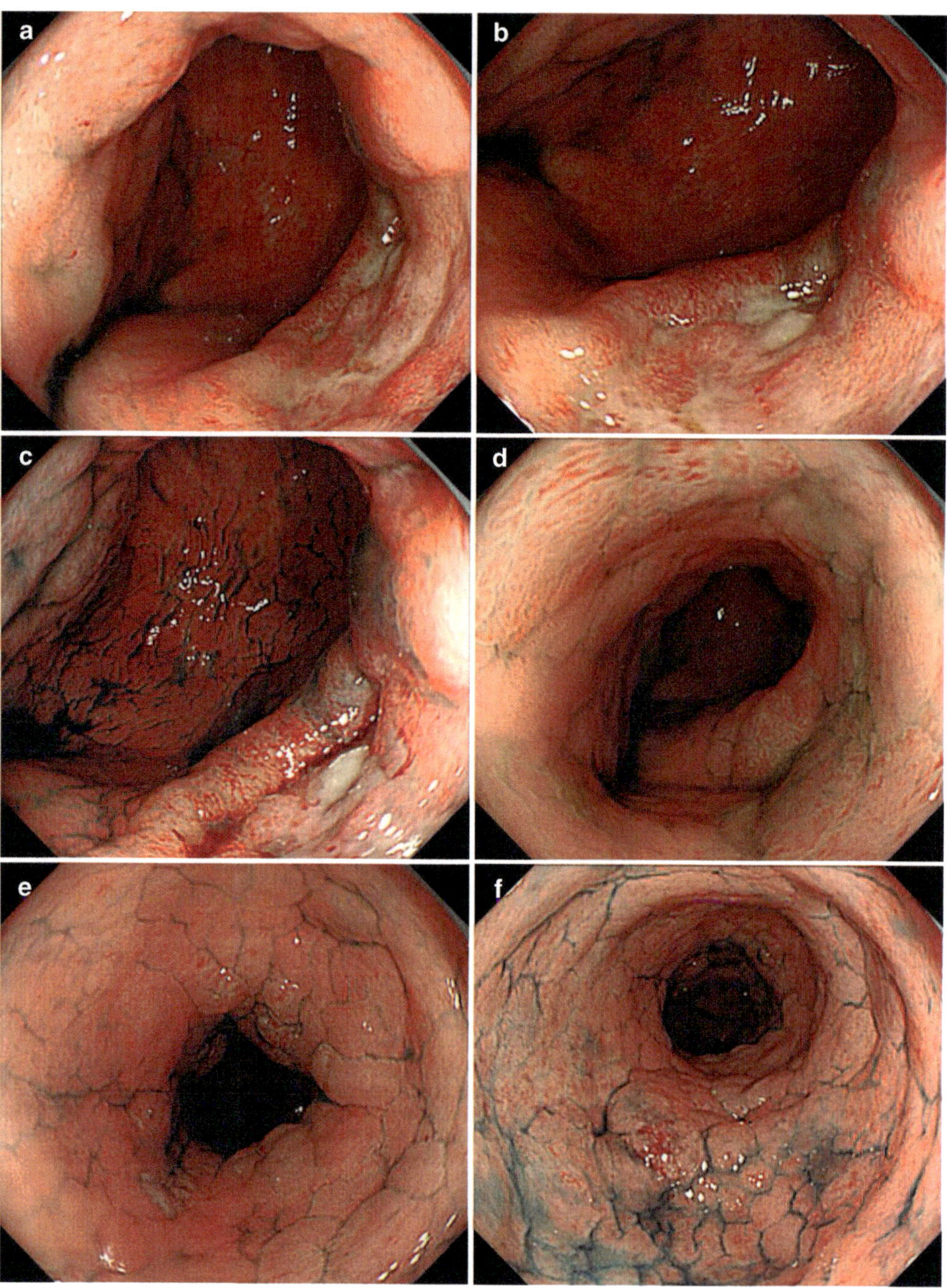

Fig. 14 Colonoscopic findings. (**a**–**d**) Conventional endoscopic observation showed an erythematous, irregularly elevated lesion in the descending colon, occupying half of the lumen, with irregular depressions. After application of indigo carmine dye, the border of the lesion was indistinct, and extension was poor even with air insufflating. (**e** and **f**) On the anal side of this lesion, there was a continuous narrowing of the lumen. The mucosal surface of the lesion was thickened throughout, with a low, indistinct elevated lesion

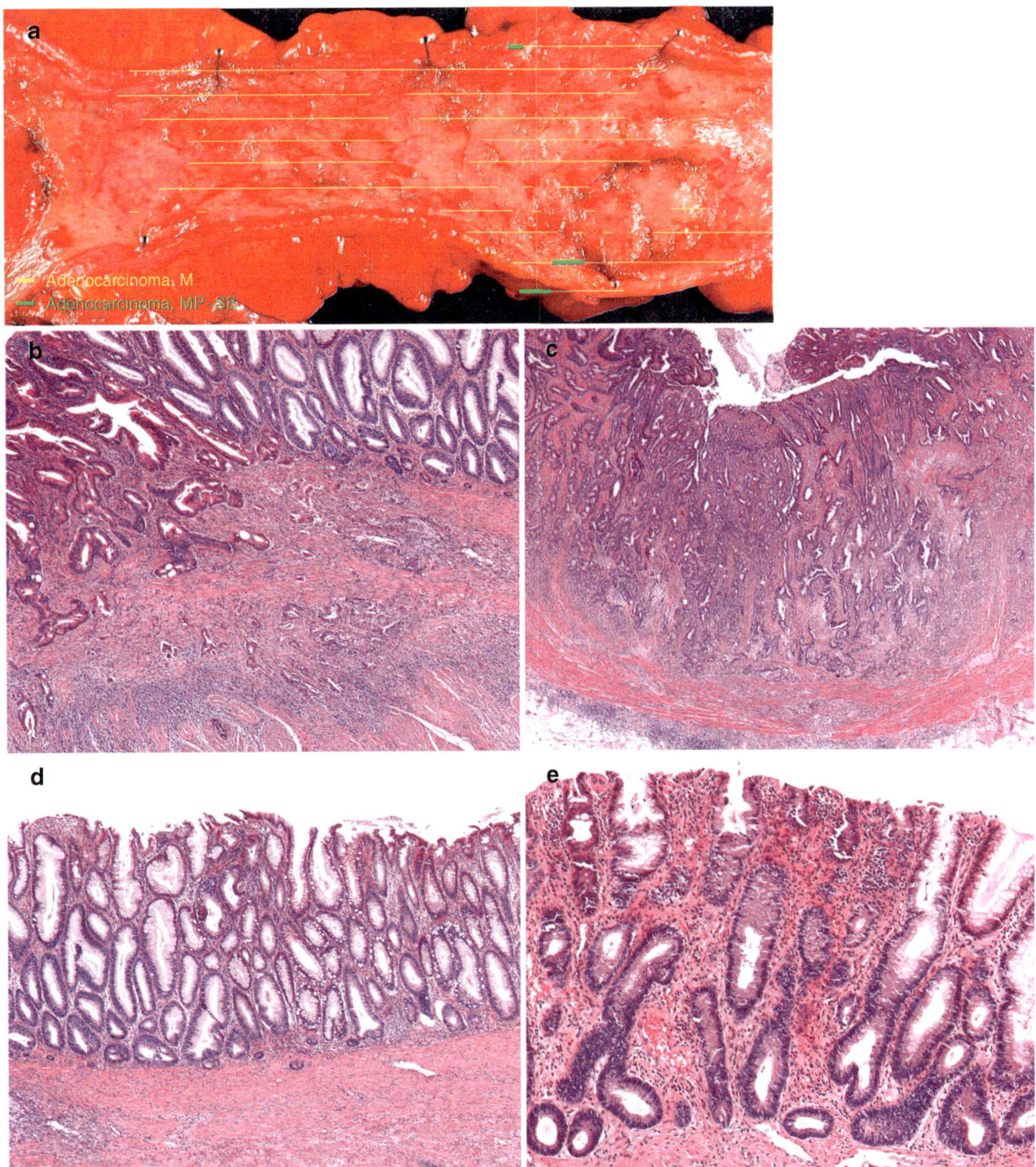

Fig. 15 Pathological image. (**a**) This is one of the multiple lesions in the same case as Case 4. The resected specimen showed a circumferential irregular mucosa extending approximately 15 cm (yellow line and green line). (**b**) Histopathologically, the lesion was characterized by extensive very well to moderately differentiated tubular adenocarcinoma. (**c**) The majority of the lesions were intramucosal with some invasion into the intrinsic muscularis propria and subserosa. (**d** and **e**) Some areas of the lesion were adenomatous (**d**) and dysplastic epithelium (**e**)

Pathological Diagnosis

- Descending colon: Type 5, 145 mm, very well to moderately differentiated adenocarcinoma with adenomatous pattern and dysplastic epithelium, pT3 (SS), Ly1a, V0, BD1, INF a, Pn1a, pPM0, pDM0, pN0.
- Stage IIa: pT3, pN0, M0, P0, H0, R0, Cur A.

Summary of this Case

Narrowing of the lumen is a suspicious finding for cancer and requires careful observation.

8 Case 17: Advanced Cancer with Unusual Morphology

Takashi Hisabe and Hiroshi Tanabe

30s, male (11 years of illness)

Type of disease: Extensive colitis
Clinical course: Relapse-remitting type
Macroscopic type: Distinct border

History of Present Illness

When he was treated for perianal fistula, he was diagnosed with ulcerative colitis and was treated with steroids and 5-ASA.

Eleven years after the onset of the disease, he underwent colonoscopy to evaluate the activity of the disease. He was diagnosed as having colorectal cancer (Fig. 16) and underwent a total colorectal resection (Fig. 17).

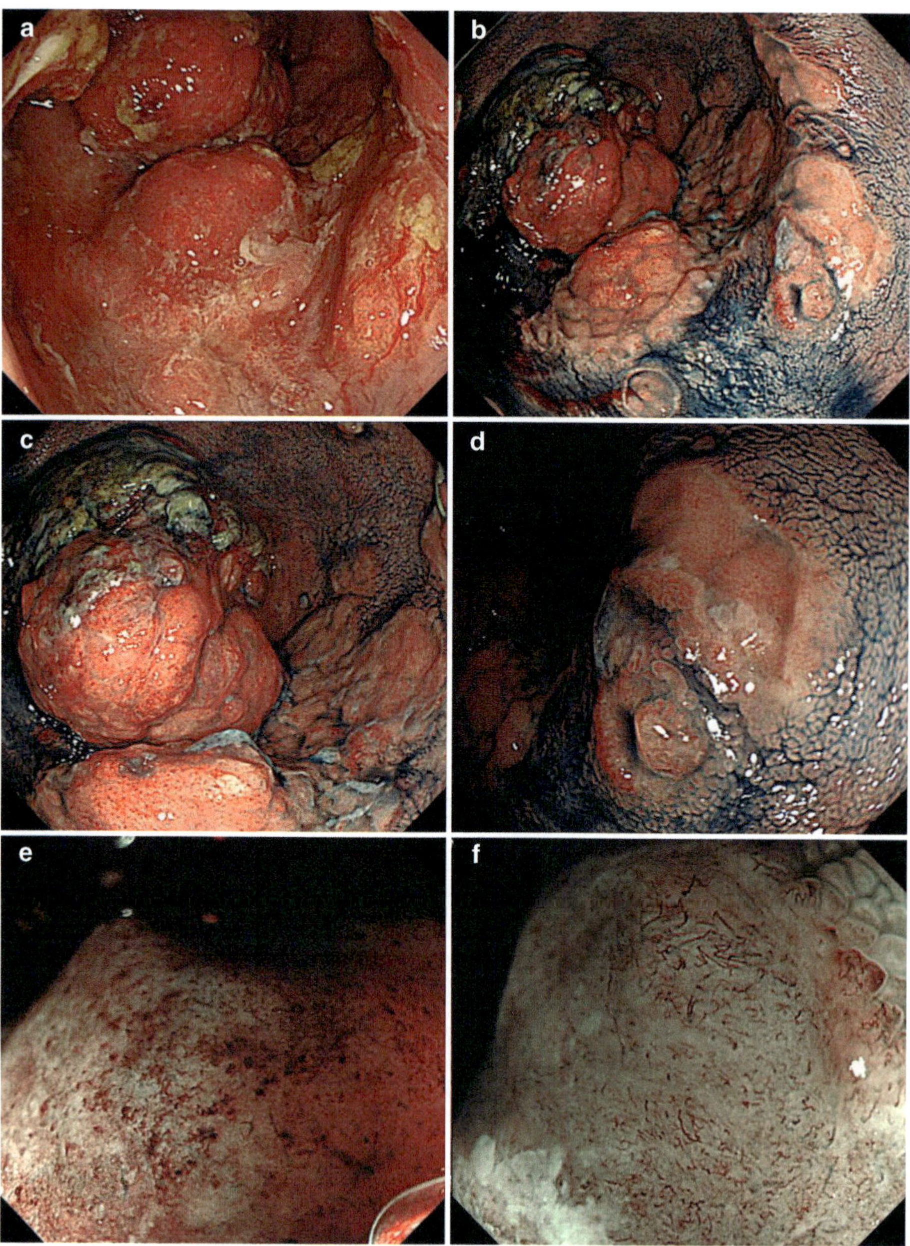

Fig. 16 Colonoscopic findings. (**a**–**d**) Conventional endoscopic examination revealed an erythematous, nodular, tall, irregularly elevated lesion in the rectum, surrounded by irregularly elevated and irregularly convex mucosal surfaces. (**e** and **f**) NBI with ME showed that the vessel pattern of the nodular and depressed lesions was irregular and asymmetrical with uneven distribution and arrangement, and the surface pattern was absent, which was a JNET classification type 3

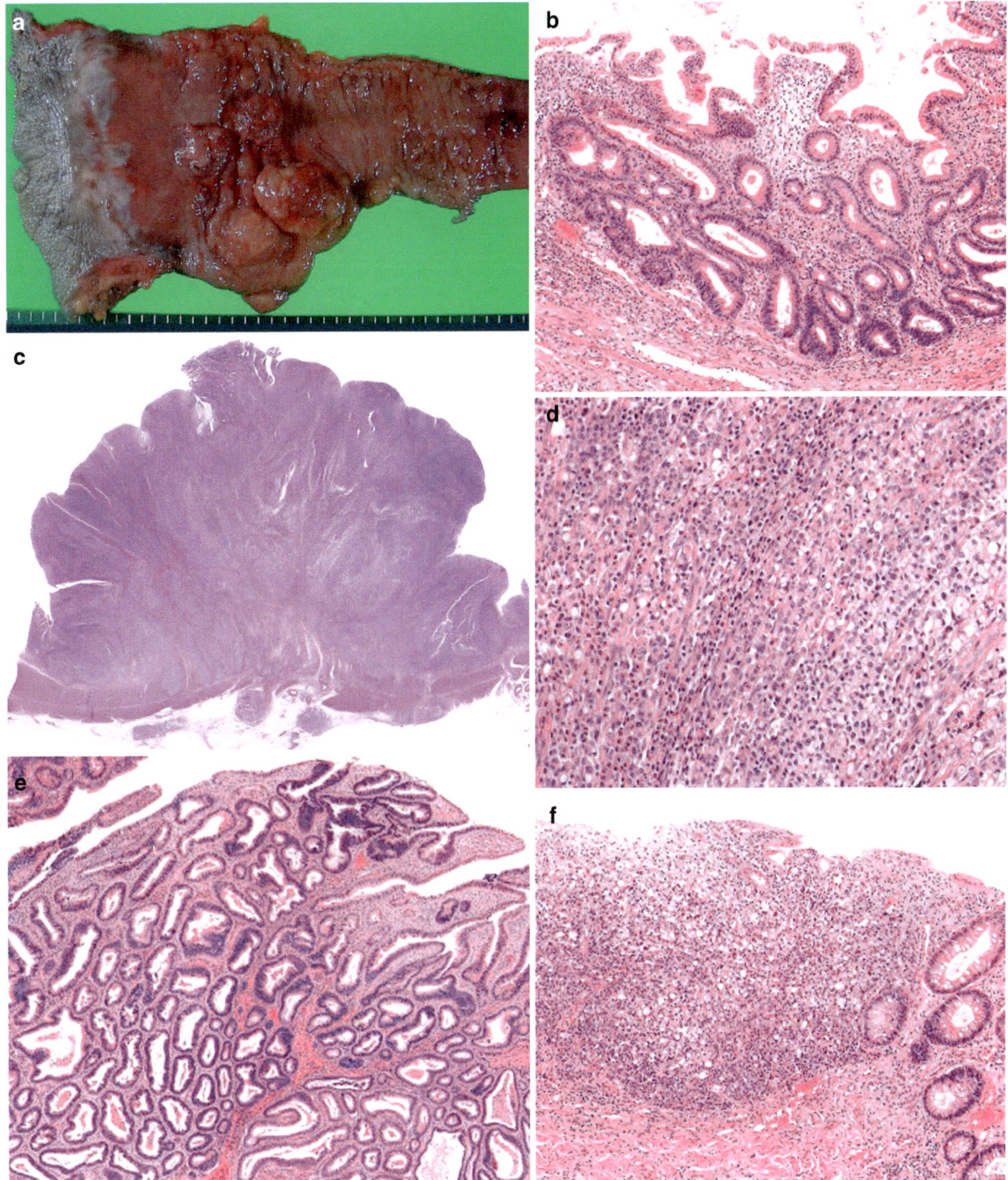

Fig. 17 Pathological image. (**a**) Multiple cancer cases. Grossly, there are multiple large and small nodular elevations in the rectum. (**b**) Histologically, around the the nodular lesion there are many foci of dysplastic epithelium in surrounding mucosa. (**c**) Lupe finding, the large, slightly whitish nodular lesion were advanced carcinoma involving the entire rectal wall. (**d**) The large, slightly whitish nodular lesion were caused by poorly differentiated adenocarcinoma. (**e**) Medium-sized, erythematous nodular lesions mainly caused by well-differentiated tubular adenocarcinoma were intramucosal carcinoma or submucosal invasion. (**f**) The hemispheric elevation was thought to be a metastatic lesion, because the histological image was similar to that of the large elevation, although it was mainly composed of poorly differentiated adenocarcinoma growing in the mucosa

Pathological Diagnosis

- Rectum : Type 1, 60×50 mm, poorly differentiated adenocarcinoma with signet-ring cells and areas of well differentiation, pT3(SS/A), Ly1c, V1a, INF c, Pn1a, pPM0, pDM0, pN2b.
- Stage IIIc : pT3, pN2b, M0, P0, H0, R0, Cur A.

Summary of this Case

Advanced cancer with unique gross morphology and histologically diverse components.

9 Case 18: Advanced Cancer in a Stenotic Area

Takashi Hisabe and Hiroshi Tanabe

30s, male (14 years of illness)

Type of disease: Extensive colitis
Clinical course: Chronic continuous type
Macroscopic type: Indistinct border

History of Present Illness

He was diagnosed with ulcerative colitis and was treated with steroids and 5-ASA.

He was then treated with steroids and leukocyte removal therapy.

Fourteen years after the onset of the disease, he underwent colonoscopy. A total circumferential stenosis was found in the descending colon, which was diagnosed as colorectal cancer by colonoscopy (Fig. 18) and by radiography (Fig. 19) and a total colorectal resection was performed (Fig. 20).

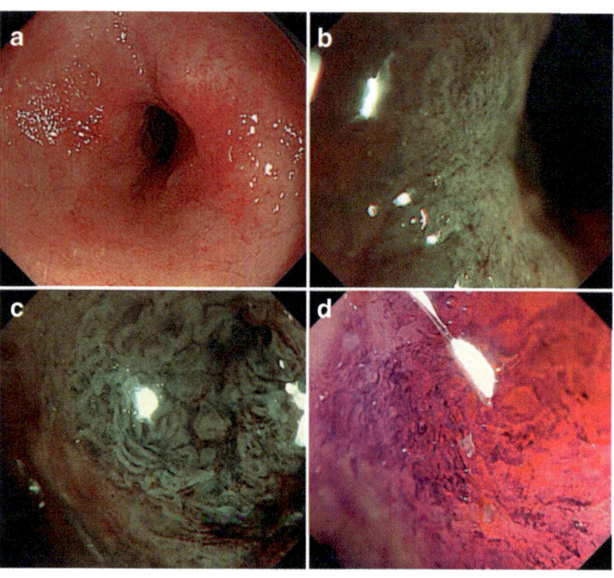

Fig. 18 Colonoscopic findings. (**a**) Conventional endoscopic observation showed a circumferential stenotic lesion in the descending colon, and the endoscope did not go through. (**b** and **c**) NBI with ME showed that the vessel pattern was nonuniform, asymmetric, and irregular in distribution and arrangement, and the surface pattern was irregular with nonuniform arcuate marginal crypt epithelium on the right side of the lesion and absent on the left side. (**d**) Pit pattern revealed a V_I-high irregularity with an indistinct pit outline and narrowing of the lumen

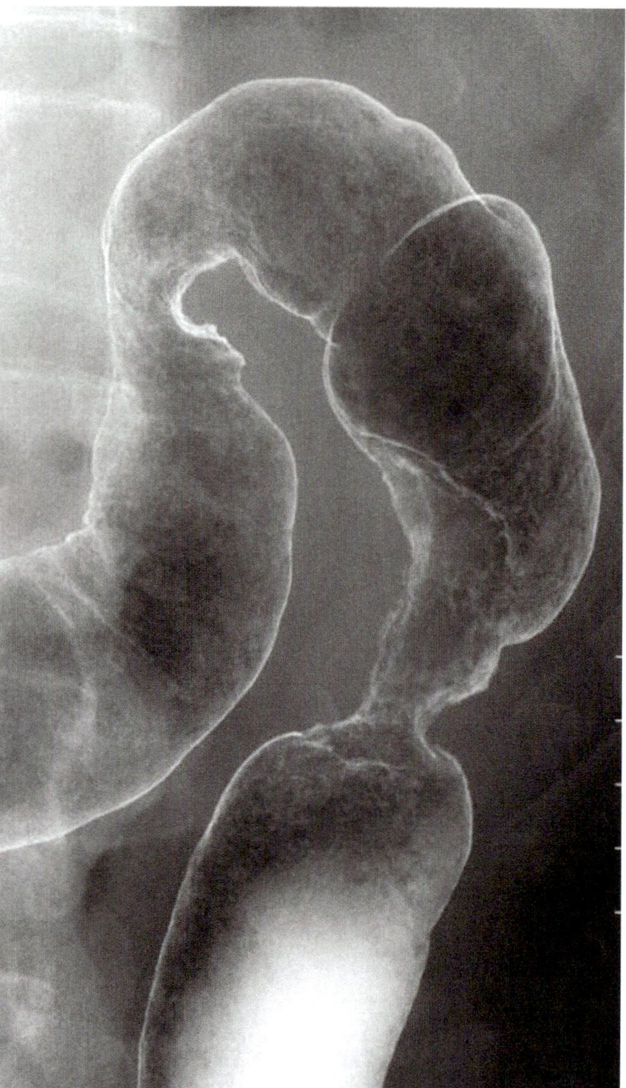

Fig. 19 Barium enema findings. Barium enema radiography showed circumferential stenosis and wall sclerosis

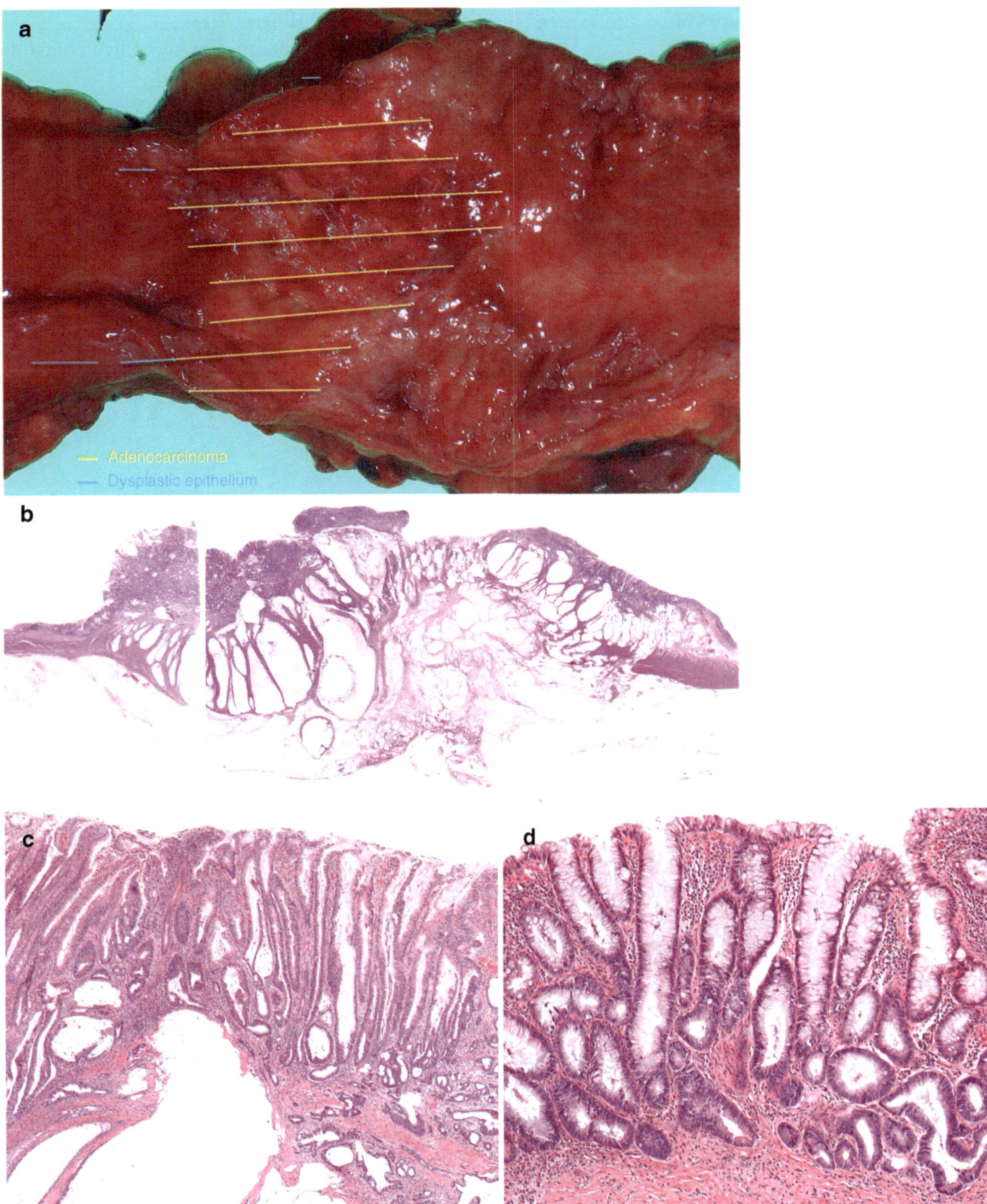

Fig. 20 Pathological image. (**a**) Grossly, a type 5 circumferential lesion was found in the stenosis of the descending colon (yellow line). (**b**) Lupe finding, the lesion was an advanced mucinous adenocarcinoma invading all layers. (**c**) Histopathologically, the lesion was very well to moderately differentiated tubular adenocarcinoma. (**d**) A part of the surrounding area dysplastic epithelium was found (**a**, blue line)

Pathological Diagnosis

- Descending colon: Type 5, 50 mm, very well to moderately differentiated adenocarcinoma with extracellular mucinous degeneration (mucinous adenocarcinoma) and dysplastic epithelium, pT4a (SE), Ly1b, V1a, BD1, INF b, Pn1a, pPM0, pDM0, pN2b.
- Stage IV: pT4a, pN2b, M0, P3, H0, R2, Cur C Lymph node metastasis and peritoneal dissemination were observed.

Summary of this Case

The findings were typical of stenosis due to advanced cancer.

10 Case 19: Advanced Cancer of the Lower Rectum

Takashi Hisabe and Hiroshi Tanabe

60s, male (30 years of illness)

Type of disease: Extensive colitis

Clinical course: Relapse-remitting type

Macroscopic type: Type 5 (indistinct border)

History of Present Illness

The patient was diagnosed with ulcerative colitis and was treated at 5-ASA.

Thirty years after the onset of the disease, a colonoscopy was performed and an irregular elevated lesion was found in the rectum (Fig. 21).

The patient was diagnosed with rectal cancer and underwent a total colorectal resection (Fig. 22).

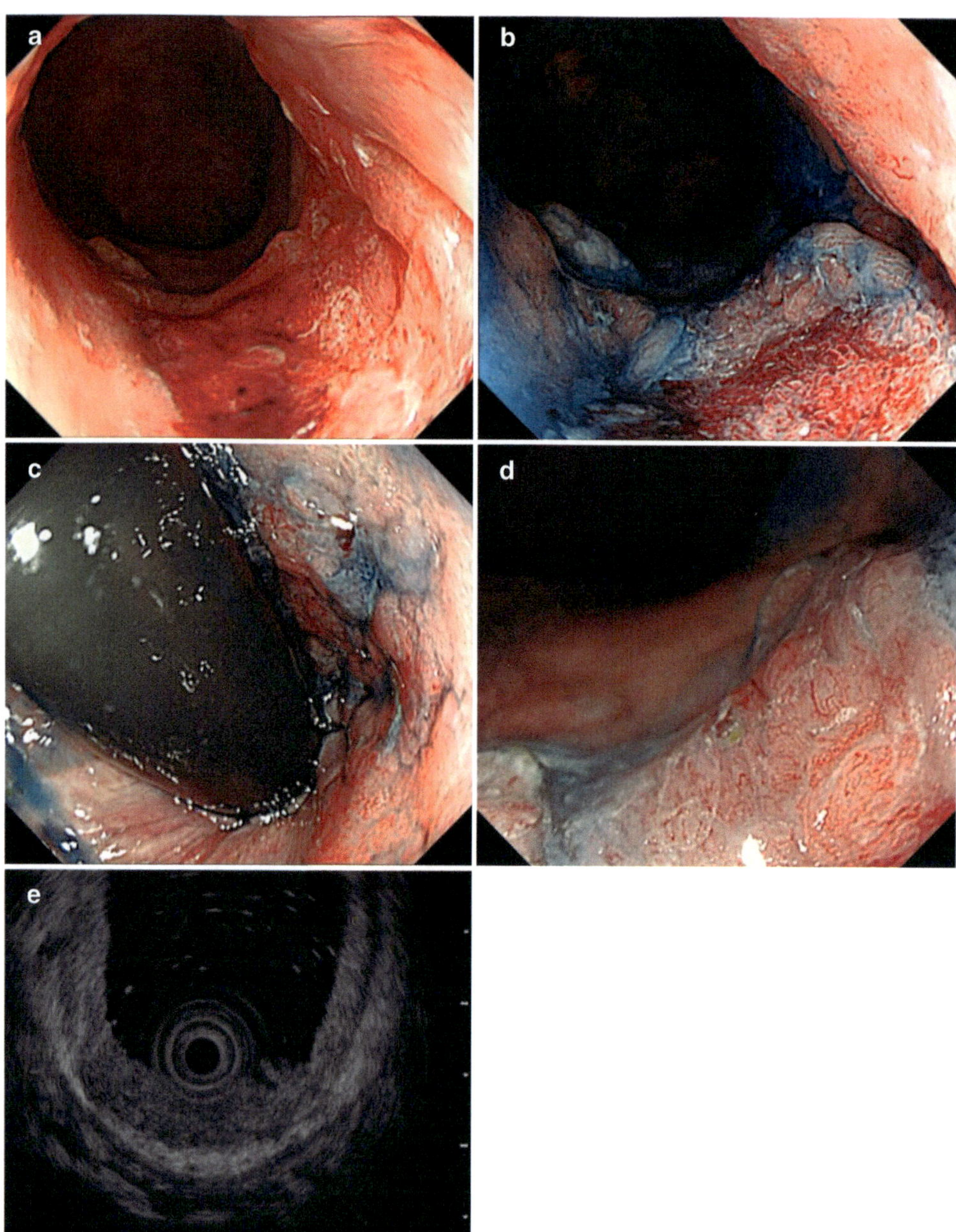

Fig. 21 Colonoscopic findings. (**a–d**) Conventional endoscopic examination revealed an erythematous, irregularly convex, raised lesion occupying 1/3 of the lumen from the lower rectum to the dentate line. Chromoendoscopy revealed a small, low-rise lesion was observed on the oral side of the lesion, with a depression on the anal side. (**e**) Ultrasonographic endoscopy revealed an irregular hypoechoic area extending deep into the third layer

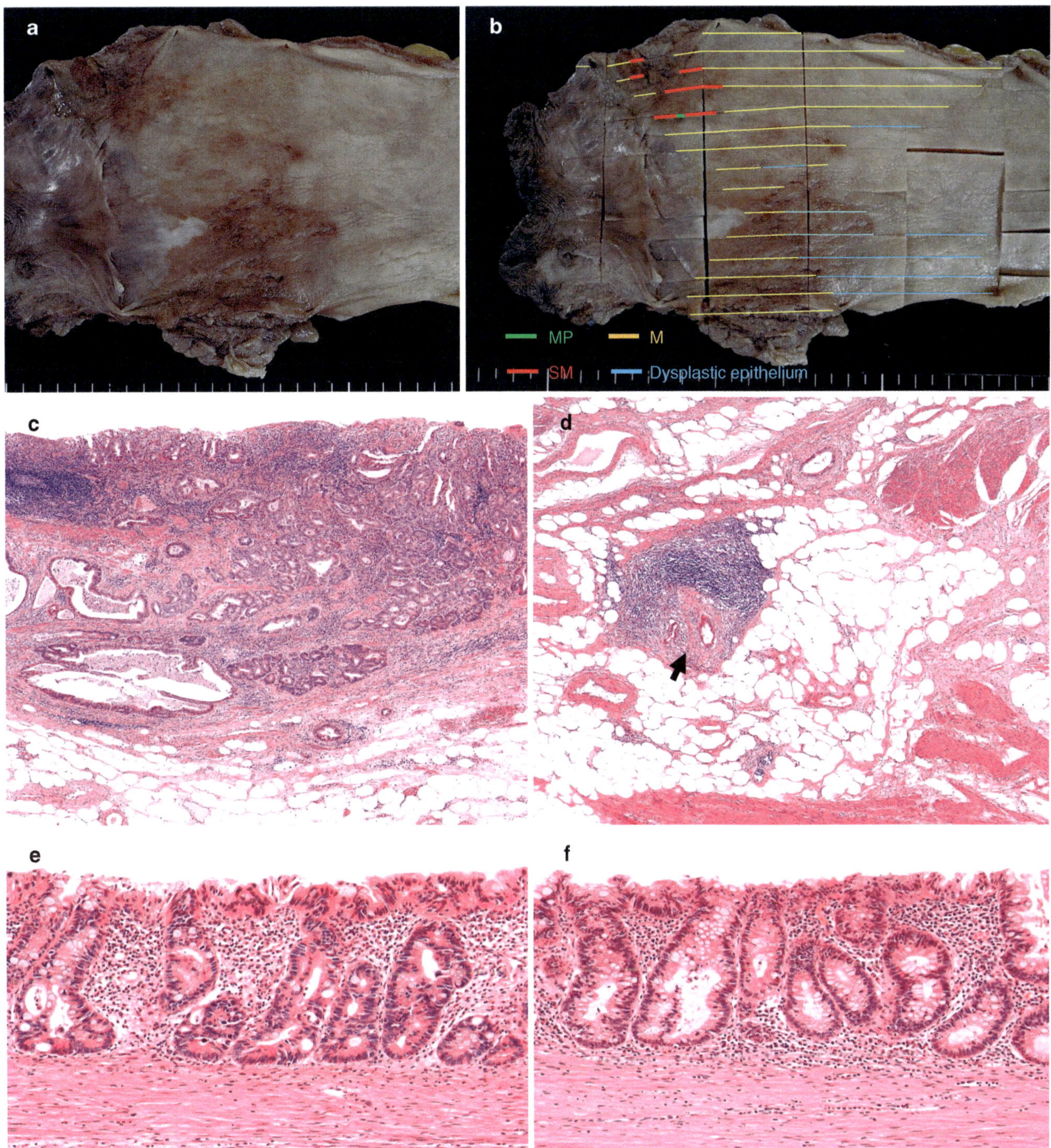

Fig. 22 Pathological image. (**a** and **b**) This is a circumferential lesion of the rectum similar to Case 13. Atrophied mucosa and some brownish mucosa were observed grossly, but macroscopically there seemed to be no evidence of advanced cancer. The majority of the lesions are intramucosal carcinomas (yellow line). (**c**) Some areas have massive invasion into the submucosa (**b**, red line). (**d**) A few carcinomatous glands are seen in the stroma between the proper muscle layers (arrow) (**b**, green line). (**e** and **f**) A dysplastic epithelium (**f**) (**b**, blue line) is present on the oral side in continuity with the carcinoma (**e**), making the diagnosis difficult

Pathological Diagnosis

- Rectum: Type 5, 130 mm, well to moderately differentiated adenocarcinoma with dysplastic epithelium, pT2 (MP), Ly1b, V1a, BD1, INF b, Pn0, pPM0, pDM0, pN 1a.
- Stage IIIa: pT2, pN1a, M0, P0, H0, R0, Cur A.

Summary of this Case

Advanced carcinoma in Rb, where a relatively difficult lesion to detect.

11 Case 20: Advanced Cancer of the Rectum

Keisuke Kawasaki, Makoto Eizuka, Tamotsu Sugai and Takayuki Matsumoto

50-years-old male (disease duration: 8 years)

Type of disease: total colitis

Clinical course: chronic persistent type

Macroscopic type: Sessile type (distinct border)

History of Present Illness

He had diarrhea, anemia, and weight loss in his 50s. He was diagnosed with ulcerative colitis of the total colitis type and received medical treatment (5-ASA and steroids). Since then, the patient has been steroid-dependent. In the surveillance colonoscopy (Fig. 23) and radiography (Fig. 24), advanced cancer was found in the rectum, and the patient underwent total colorectal resection and ileostomy (Fig. 25).

Based on the findings of radiography, conventional endoscopy, and magnifying endoscopy, the lesion was considered to be an advanced carcinoma, and surgical resection was performed.

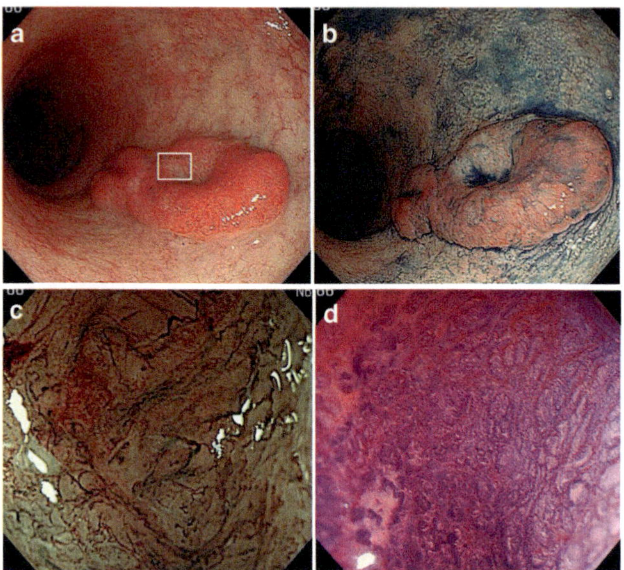

Fig. 23 Colonoscopic findings. (**a**) There is a protruding lesion with erythematous tone containing depression in the upper rectum. It is tense and had converging folds on the oral side. (**b**) Dye-spread image. The borders and superficial depressions are more distinct. There are no dysplasias in the surrounding area of the tumor. (**c**) Magnifying endoscopic image with NBI of the white box in (**a**). The structure had disappeared and irregular dilated vessels are seen. (**d**) Magnifying chromoendoscopic image with the use of crystal violet solutions of the white box in (**a**). Small irregular pits are densely observed

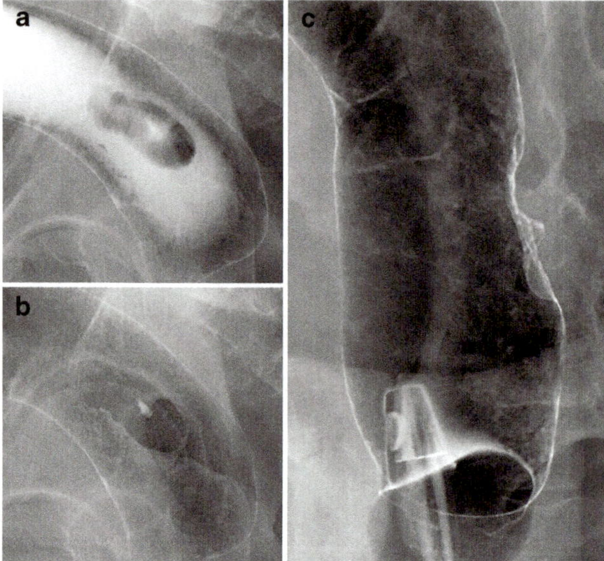

Fig. 24 Findings of barium enema examination. (**a**) There is a protruding lesion on the right wall of the upper rectum. There are barium spots on the surface, and the presence of a depression is suspected. (**b**) Double-contrast radiography reveals the lesion of a protruding lesion with a smooth surface and a depressed area. (**c**) Wall rigidity under the profile view at the lesion is present

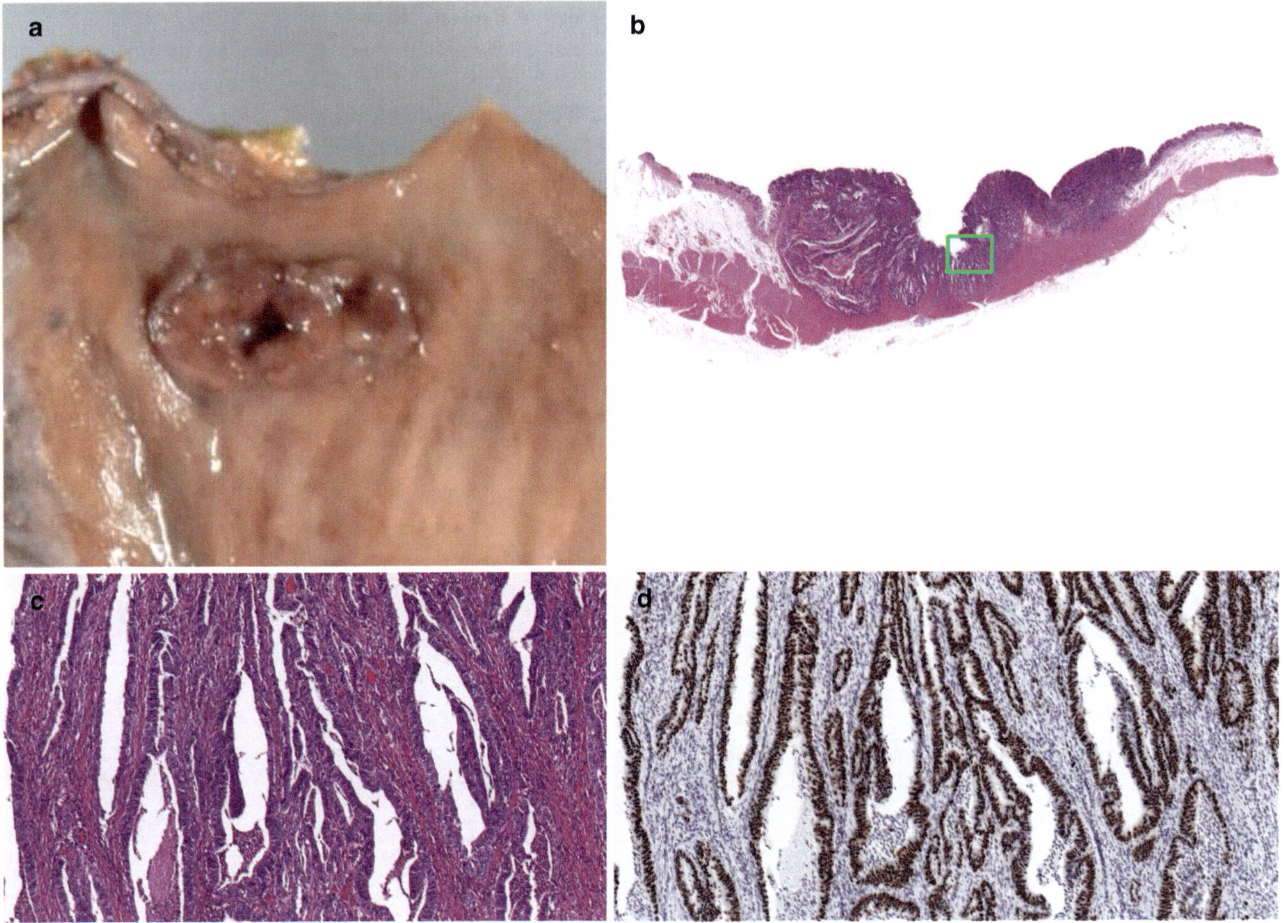

Fig. 25 Pathological image. (**a**) Resection specimen. There is a protruding lesion with a central depression, 34 × 22 mm in size, in the rectum. (**b**) Loupe image. There is no dysplasia in the surrounding mucosa, and the tumor cells have invaded the proper muscle layer. (**c**) Magnified image of green box in (**b**) (H.E. staining). The tumor area shows well-differentiated to moderately differentiated tubular adenocarcinoma. (**d**) P53 staining image in the green box of b. P53 is strongly positive in the tumor area

Pathological Diagnosis

- Rectum: Type 2, 34 × 22 mm, well to moderately differentiated adenocarcinoma, pT2 (MP), Ly1, V1, pPM0, pDM0, pN0. Stage I: pT2, pN0, M0, P0, H0, R0.

Summary of this Case

The tumor was located in the affected area of ulcerative colitis, and there was no dysplasia in the surrounding area, but P53 was highly positive in the tumor area, suggesting a UC-associated tumor. Barium enema and colonoscopy showed that the depth of the tumor was not difficult to diagnose.

12 Case 21: Advanced Cancer with Good Extension

Keisuke Kawasaki, Makoto Eizuka, Tamotsu Sugai and Takayuki Matsumoto

30-years-old male (disease duration: 8 years)

Type of disease: total colitis

Clinical course: unknown

Macroscopic type: Superficial elevated type (distinct border)

History of Present Illness

He had intermittent upper abdominal pain in his 20s but neglected it. In his 30s, he had back pain, jaundice, anemia and was diagnosed with primary sclerosing cholangitis and ulcerative colitis. Subsequently, He was treated with 5-ASA and steroid. One year later, a surveillance colonoscopy showed an elevated lesion in the ascending colon (Fig. 26), and a living donor liver transplant and right hemicolectomy were performed (Fig. 27).

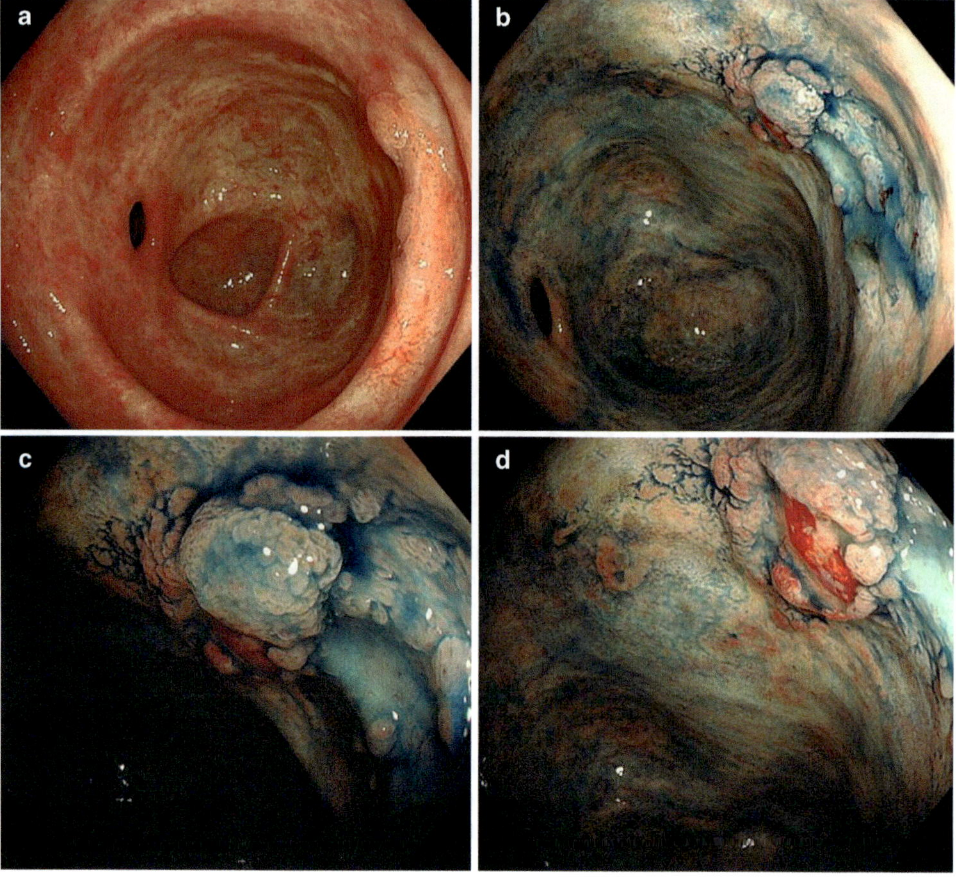

Fig. 26 Colonoscopic findings. (**a**) There is an elevated lesion with the same color tone as the surrounding mucosa in the ascending colon. Although the background mucosa has abnormal vascularization, there is no obvious erosion or ulceration, indicating ulcerative colitis in remission. (**b**) Dye-spread image. The border is clear, and extension under air-insufflation is good, but there is a mild convergence at the oral side. There is no evidence of dysplasia around the tumor. (**c**) A high elevation with a villous surface is present at the oral side. (**d**) An area of depression with easily hemorrhagic tendency is present on the oral side of an elevation shown in (**b**). Surgical resection was performed because the deep submucosal invasion was suspected due to the above findings

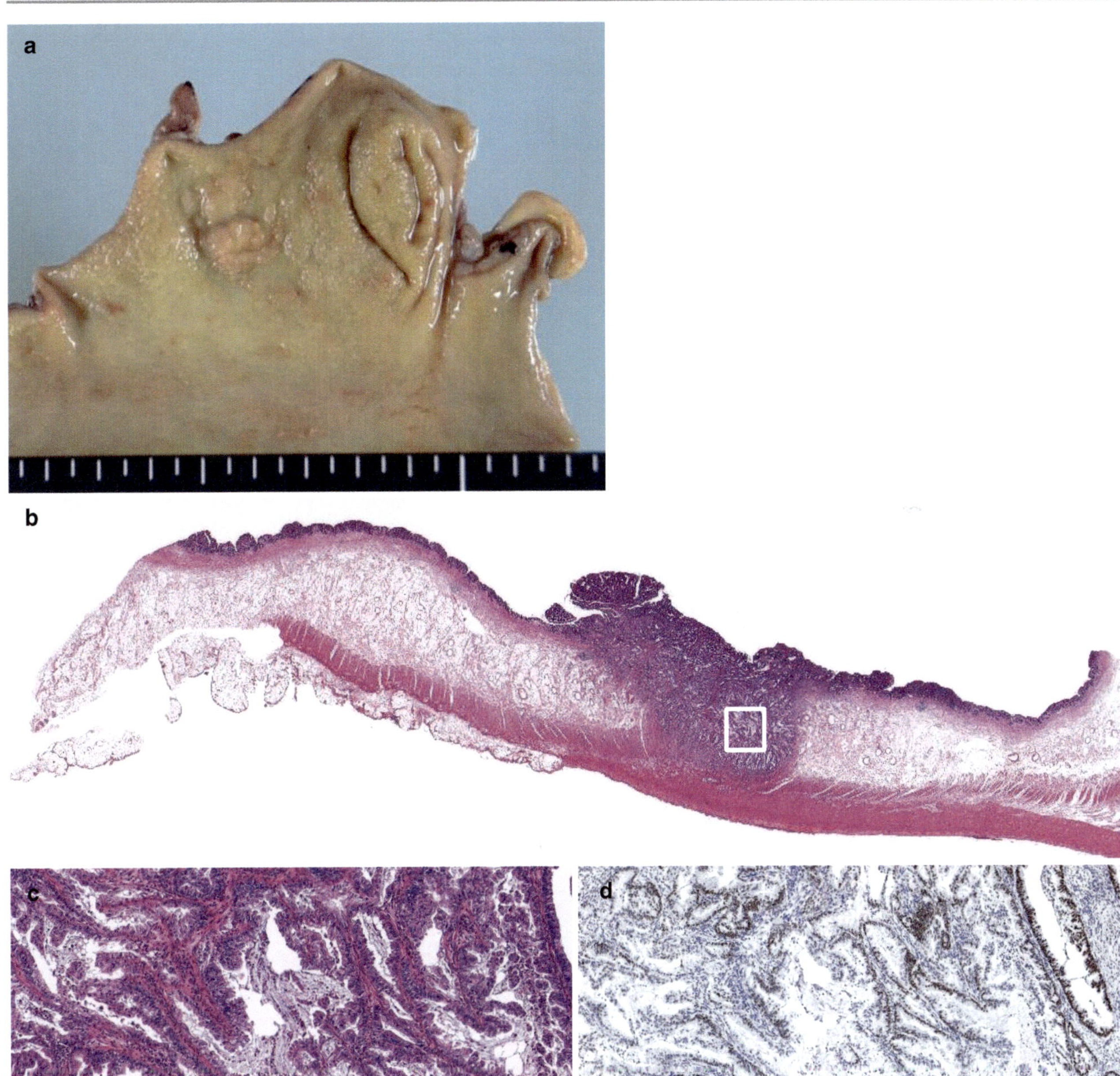

Fig. 27 Pathological image. (**a**) Resected specimen. There is a flat-elevated lesion, 23 × 21 mm in size, in the ascending colon. (**b**) Loupe image. There is no dysplasia in the surrounding mucosa, and the tumor cells invaded the proper muscular layer. (**c**) Enlarged image of the white box of (**b**) (H.E. staining). The tumor area shows moderately to well-differentiated tubular adenocarcinoma. (**d**) P53 staining image. p53 is strongly positive in the tumor area

Pathological Diagnosis

- Ascending colon: Type 5, 23 × 21 mm, well to moderately differentiated adenocarcinoma, pT2 (MP), Ly2, V0, pHM0, pVM0, pN0. Stage I: pT2, pN0, M0, P0, H0, R0.

Summary of this Case

This patient had primary sclerosing cholangitis. Because the tumor was located in the affected area of ulcerative colitis, and was also positive for P53, we diagnosed it as UC-associated neoplasia. Because the tumor was a elevated lesion with a clear depression and relatively good extension under air-insufflation, the depth of invasion was considered as a deep submucosal invasion. However, it invaded the proper muscular layer. This case was deeper than expected.

Part III

Cases of CD Associated Cancers

Small Intestinal Cancer: 5 Cases

Kitaro Futami, Hiroshi Tanabe, Keisuke Kawasaki,
Koji Ikegami, Minako Fujiwara, and Takayuki Matsumoto

K. Futami (✉)
Center for Clinical Medical Research (Surgery), Fukuoka University Chikushi Hospital, Chikushino, Japan

H. Tanabe
Department of Pathology, Fukuoka University Chikushi Hospital, Chikushino, Japan

K. Kawasaki
Department of Gastroenterology, Iwate Medical University, Iwate, Japan

Department of Medicine and Clinical Science, Graduate School of Medical Sciences, Kyushu University, Fukuoka, Japan

K. Ikegami
Department of Medicine and Clinical Science, Graduate School of Medical Sciences, Kyushu University, Fukuoka, Japan

M. Fujiwara
Department of Pathology, National Hospital Organization Kyushu Medical Center, Fukuoka, Japan

T. Matsumoto
Department of Gastroenterology, Iwate Medical University, Iwate, Japan

T. Matsui et al. (eds.), *Atlas of Inflammatory Bowel Disease-Associated Intestinal Cancer*,
https://doi.org/10.1007/978-981-19-3413-1_8

1 Case 1: Early Cancer of the Ileum Diagnosed by Endoscopic Surveillance

Kitaro Futami and Hiroshi Tanabe

40s, male, SL type, 26 years of illness

Onset as a teen with abdominal pain and diagnosed as CD. In the same year, he underwent ileocecal resection. In his 30s, he was referred to our hospital for refractory perianal abscess. After seton drainage, an immunomodulator and biologic agent were introduced against intestinal flare-up. Four years later, remission was achieved, but anorectal stenosis occurred as a complication. Thereafter anal dilation therapy under anesthesia was repeated, and endoscopic surveillance for cancer was performed. Five years later, atypical epithelium was detected in the reddish polyp at the oral side of the ileocolonic anastomosis and in the surrounding mucosa, and atypical epithelium was detected by three successive biopsies (Fig. 1), so he underwent surgery. Small bowel radiography and computed tomography detected no neoplastic lesion. CEA value: 1.7 ng/mL.

Surgery

Ileocolonic resection, lymph node dissection, end-to-end anastomosis. Resected 10 cm from the anal side and 10 cm from the oral side (total 20 cm resection).

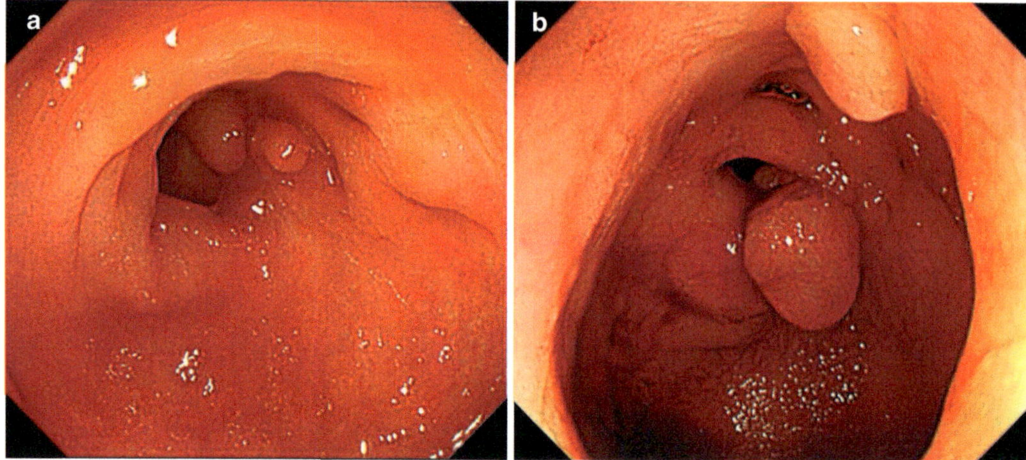

Fig. 1 Colonoscopy findings: (**a**) Two erythematous polypoid lesions at the oral side of the ileocolonic anastomosis. (**b**) Even in close-up view, no suspicious findings of atypia in the surrounding mucosa were noted, but atypical epithelium was detected by a biopsy

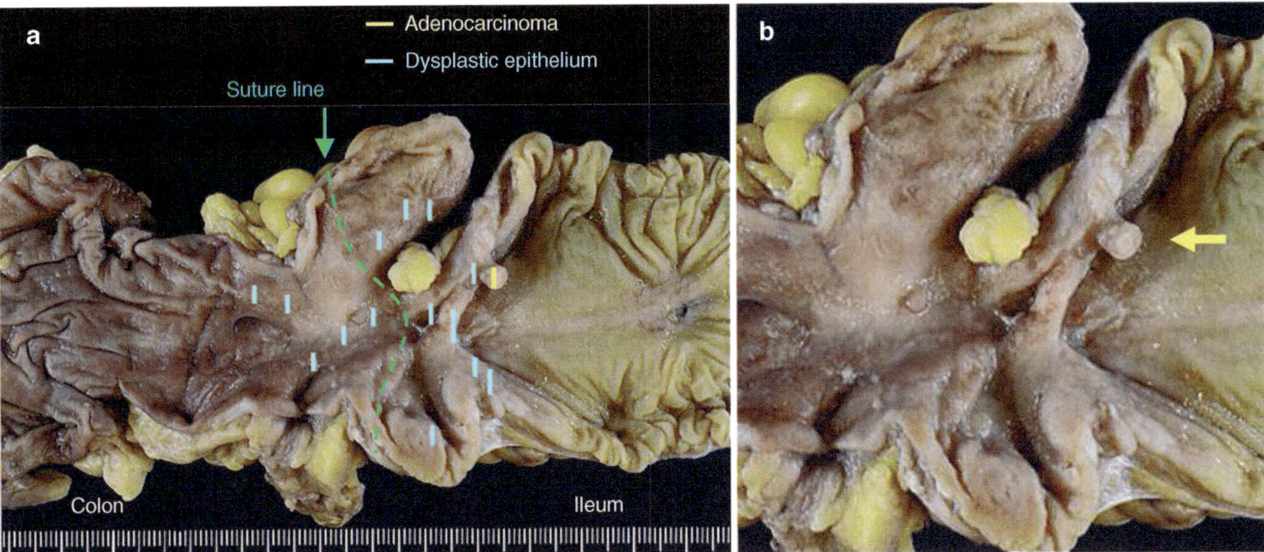

Fig. 2 Gross finding of the resected specimen: (**a**) Area of histological difference was shown by colored lines. There was a polypoid lesion (A 6-mm in size, yellow line) at the ileocolonic anastomosis (green arrow). Yellow line shows adenocarcinoma and blue line shows area of dysplastic epithelium with mild atypia around the ileocolonic anastomosis. (**b**) Close-up view of cancer (yellow arrow)

Fig. 3 Loupe image: There were scattered areas composed of very well-differentiated carcinoma and the tumor cells invaded all the mucosal layer

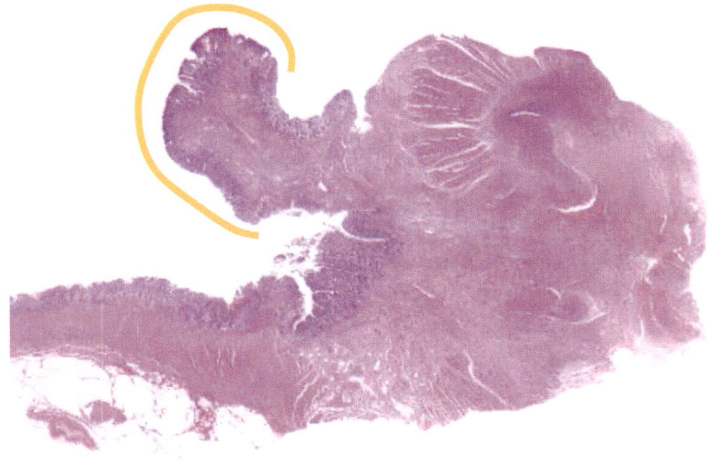

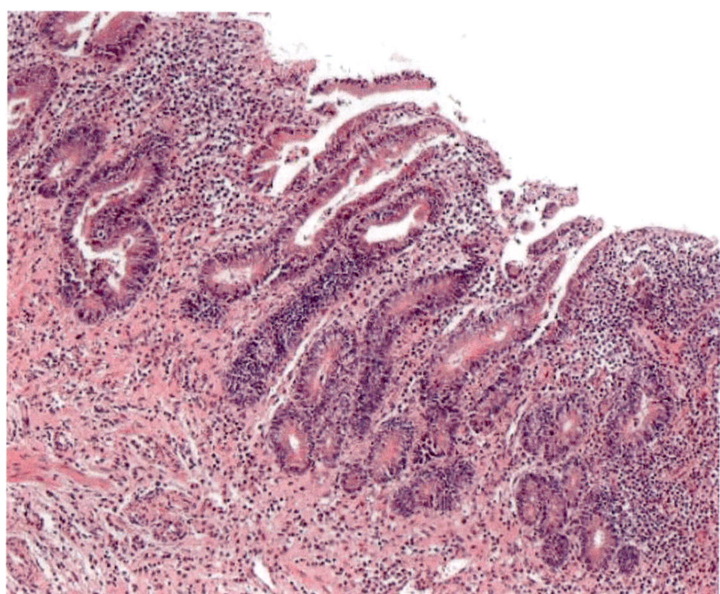

Fig. 4 H.E. staining of the adenocarcinoma: Histology of the polypoid lesion showing a very well-differentiated tubular adenocarcinoma

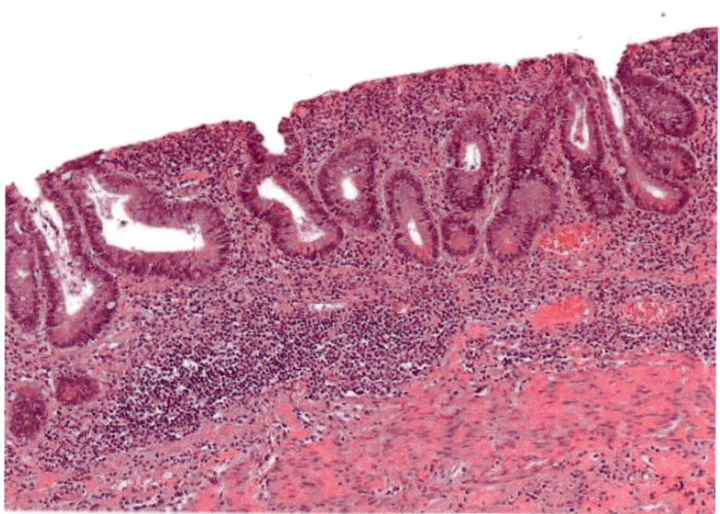

Fig. 5 H.E. staining of the dysplastic epithelium: Histology of the dysplastic epithelium in the surrounding mucosa. It was difficult to determine whether it was regenerative or neoplastic, and it was difficult to recognize grossly

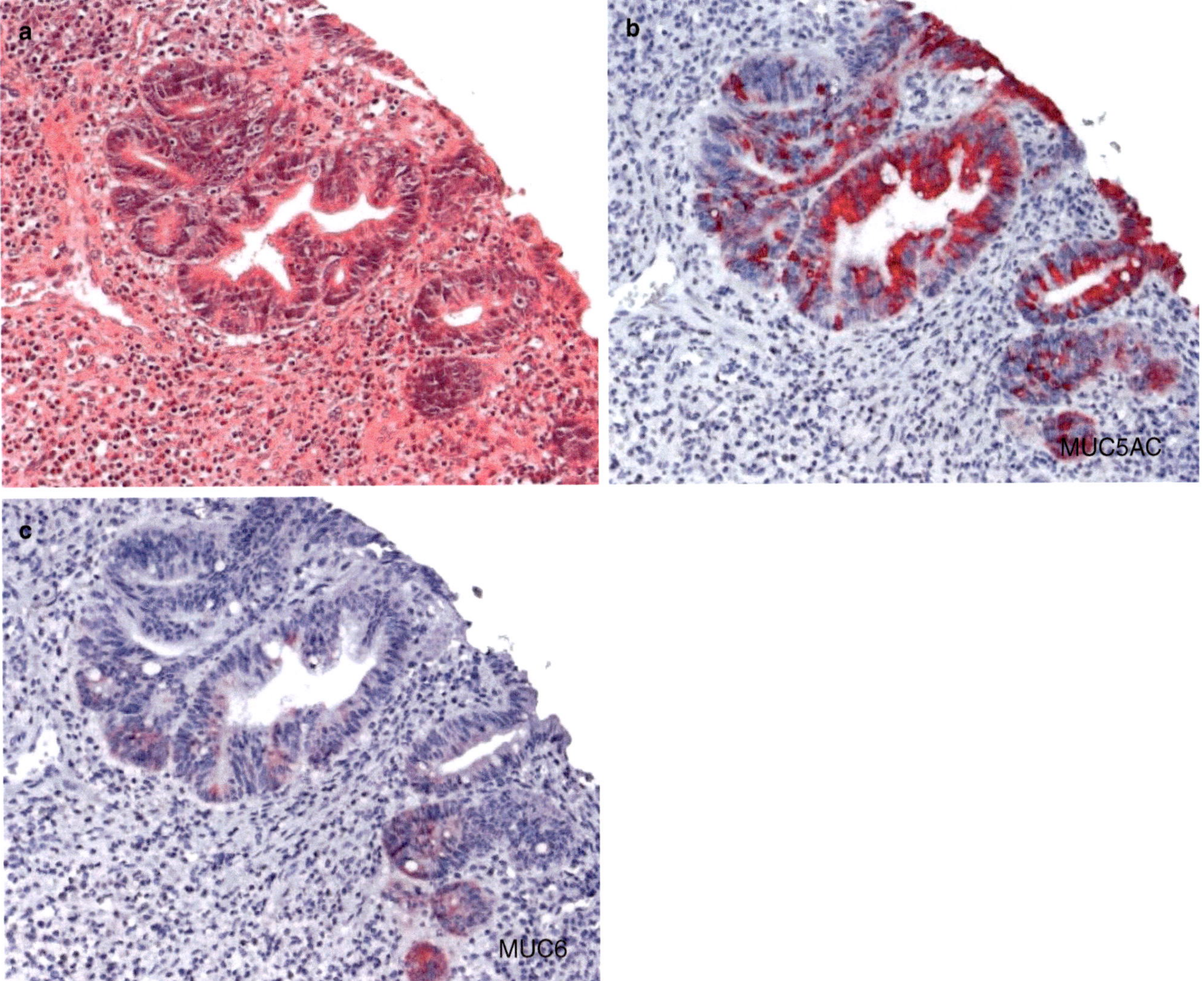

Fig. 6 H.E. and immunohistochemical staining of the adenocarcinoma: (**a**) H.E. staining of the adenocarcinoma. (**b** and **c**) MUC5AC (**b**) and MUC6 (**c**) staining was partly positive for tumor cells, indicating a mixed gastric mucin phenotype

The Pathological Diagnosis

- Ileum: Type 0-Ip, 6 mm, very well-differentiated adenocarcinoma with dysplastic epithelium, pTis (M), Ly0, V0, BD1, INF a, pPM0, pDM0, pN0 (Figs. 2, 3, 4, 5, and 6)
- Stage 0: pTis, pN0, M0, H0, R0, Cur A.

Summary

Concerning dysplastic epithelium there are diagnostic problems in not only UC but also in CD. Atypical glandular ducts surrounding the main lesion are often present (Figs. 2 and 5). However, most of the dysplastic epitheliums are modified by strong background inflammation and it is difficult to determine whether they are regenerative or neoplastic clearly.

When performing colonoscopy, observation up to the ileum and a proactive biopsy are necessary for surveillance.

2 Case 2: Multiple Ileal Carcinomas Diagnosed During Operation for Intestinal Obstruction

Kitaro Futami and Hiroshi Tanabe

30s, female, SL type, 16 years of illness

Onset in her 20s with ileus diagnosed 3 years later as CD with type I diabetes mellitus on insulin use. She underwent exclusion bypass and strictureplasty. No medical treatment was delivered for 10 years after intestinal surgery; however, she was hospitalized because of ileus due to multiple stenoses caused by recurrent lesions and underwent emergent surgery. Two cancer lesions were diagnosed by intraoperative findings and pathology (Fig. 7a, b). No evidence of neoplastic lesion was noted on small bowel radiography or computed tomography. CEA value: 2.1 ng/mL, CA19-9 value: 962 u/mL.

Surgery

Partial ileal resection, lymph node dissection, end-to-end anastomosis, with an intraoperative rapid pathological diagnosis (well-differentiated adenocarcinoma)

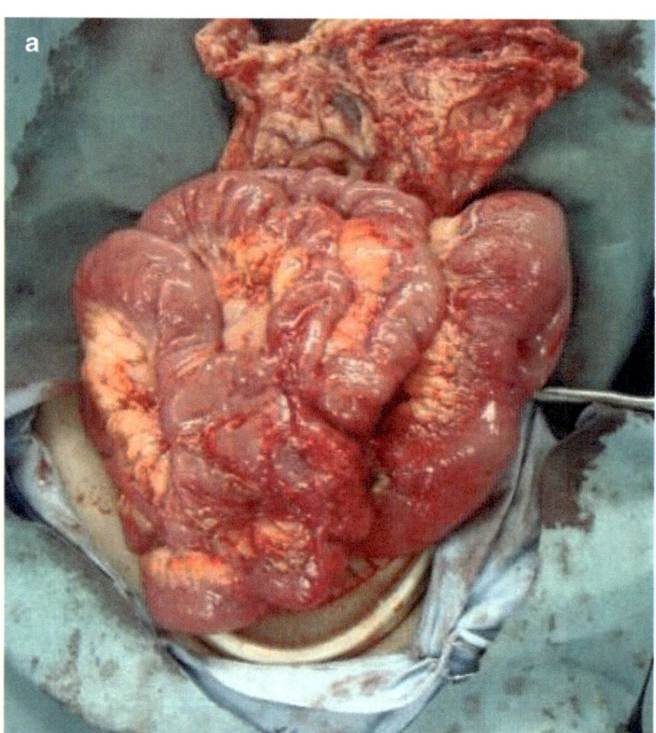

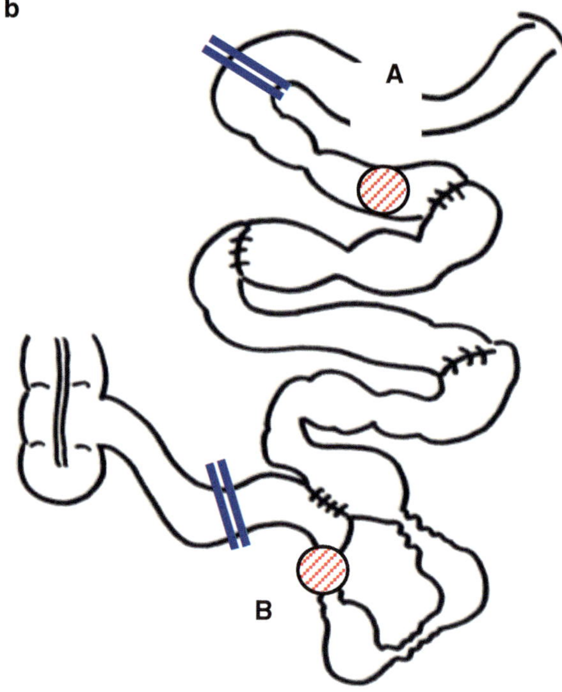

Fig. 7 (**a**) Intraoperative findings: Confirmation of disseminated lesions at laparotomy. While exploring the diseased intestine, the whole intestine was palpated as a single mass. (**b**) A schematic illustration of the location of the two lesions: One is located at previous stenotic site (A) and one is located at the blind loop intestine by exclusion bypass (B)

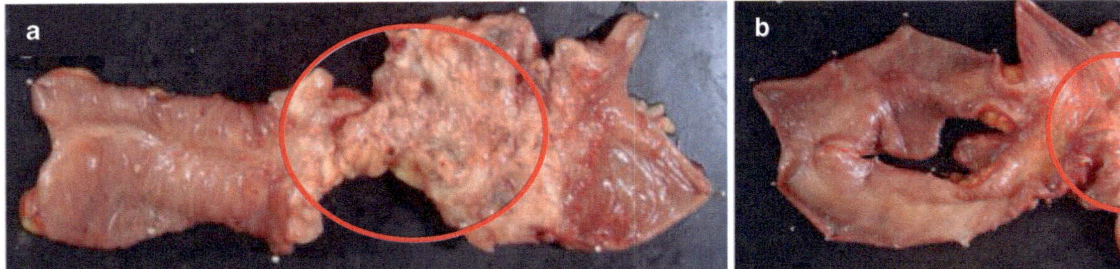

Fig. 8 Macroscopic findings: Total circumferential stricture with irregular ulcerative lesion in the ileum (lesion A, **a**), and an elevated lesion with central ulcer in the blind loop (lesion B, **b**)

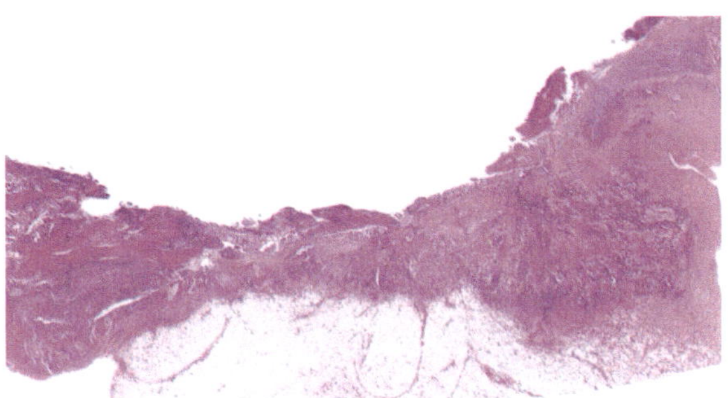

Fig. 9 Lupe image of lesion A: The oral ileal lesion (lesion A) was a tumor occupying the entire circumference of the intestine almost coincident with the faded area (gross picture Fig. 8a)

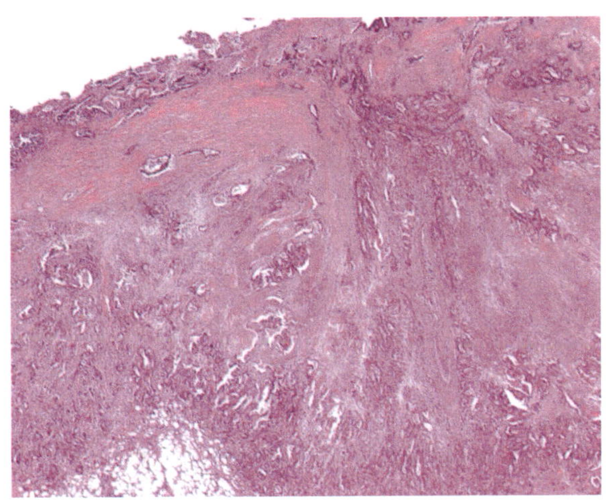

Fig. 10 Histologic picture of lesion A: The type 3 advanced carcinoma with extensive whole-thickness invasion and ulceration of well- to moderately differentiated tubular adenocarcinoma

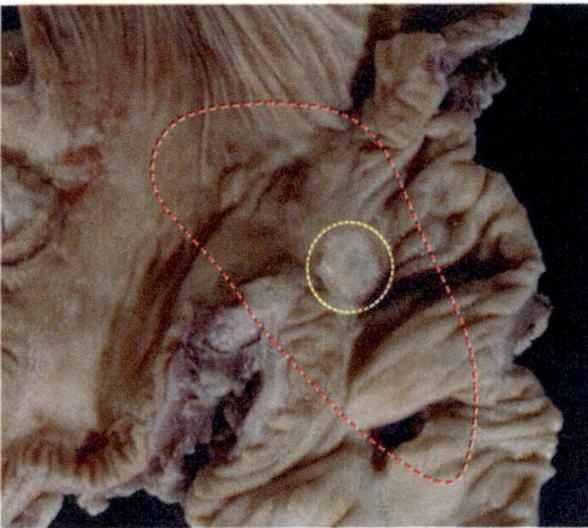

Fig. 11 Gross finding of lesion B: The lesion on the anal side (lesion B) which was located near the lateral anastomosis of the intestine by bypass surgery. Small intramucosal lesions and superficial exposure of submucosal carcinoma can be seen in the yellow circle, but most of the tumor appeared to have spread through the surrounding submucosa and subserosa, as shown with the red line

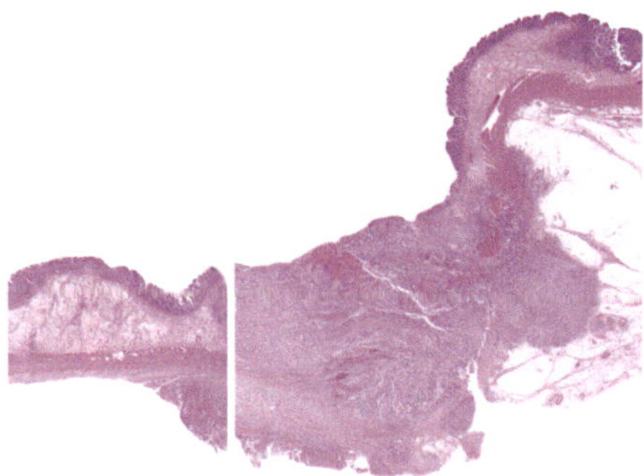

Fig. 12 Lupe image of lesion B: The anal ileal lesion (lesion B) was mainly well- to moderately differentiated tubular adenocarcinoma with areas of poor differentiation and type 3 advanced carcinoma involving the whole thickness of the ileal wall

The Pathological Diagnosis

- Oral ileal lesion (A): Type 3, 120 mm, well- to moderately differentiated adenocarcinoma, pT4a (SE), Ly1c, V1a, BD1, Pn1b, pPM0, pDM0, pN2a.
- Anal ileal lesion (B): Type 3, 80 × 40 mm, well- to moderately differentiated adenocarcinoma with areas of poor differentiation, pT4a (SE), Ly1c, V1a, BD2, Pn1b, pPM0, pDM0, pN2a.
- Stage IV: pT4a, pN2a, M0, P3, H0, R2, Cur C.

Summary

- Two advanced ileal cancers causing ileus were found in a patient who ceased any medical treatment for a long time. The oral lesion (lesion A) was a tumor occupying the entire circumference of the intestine almost coincident with the faded area (gross picture, Fig. 8a) and was a type 3 advanced carcinoma (Figs. 9 and 10). The lesion on the anal side (lesion B, Figs. 8b, 11, and 12) was located near the lateral anastomosis of the intestine by bypass surgery. Both lesions showed marked lymphatic invasion, lymph node metastasis, and numerous disseminated lesions on the serosal side.

3 Case 3: Synchronous Quadruple Ileal Carcinomas Diagnosed by Postoperative Pathological Findings of Multiple Stenoses

Kitaro Futami and Hiroshi Tanabe

40s, female, SL type, 22 years of illness

Onset in her 20s with perianal lesions. Ten years later, she was diagnosed with UC. Thirteen years after the onset, she underwent emergency surgery due to ileal perforation and was diagnosed with CD. One year after surgery, she recurred and started treatment at our hospital. Nutritional therapy, immunomodulators, anal dilation using a finger or mechanical bougie were performed. Later, biologic therapy and endoscopic dilation of the ileal stricture were continued, but three biopsies at endoscopic dilation did not detect any atypical epithelium. After 7 years of treatment at our facility, she developed ileus symptoms again and was unable to undergo endoscopic dilation therapy again. Active lesions were obvious; however, no cancerous findings were detected on radiographic examination of the small intestine preoperatively (Fig. 13). CEA value: 0.9 ng/mL, CA19-9 value: 3.0 µg/mL.

Surgery

1. Partial ileal resection (53 cm including previous anastomosis) with end-to-end anastomosis.
2. Ileocolonic resection (14 cm including previous anastomosis) with end-to-end anastomosis and 170 cm of remaining small intestine.

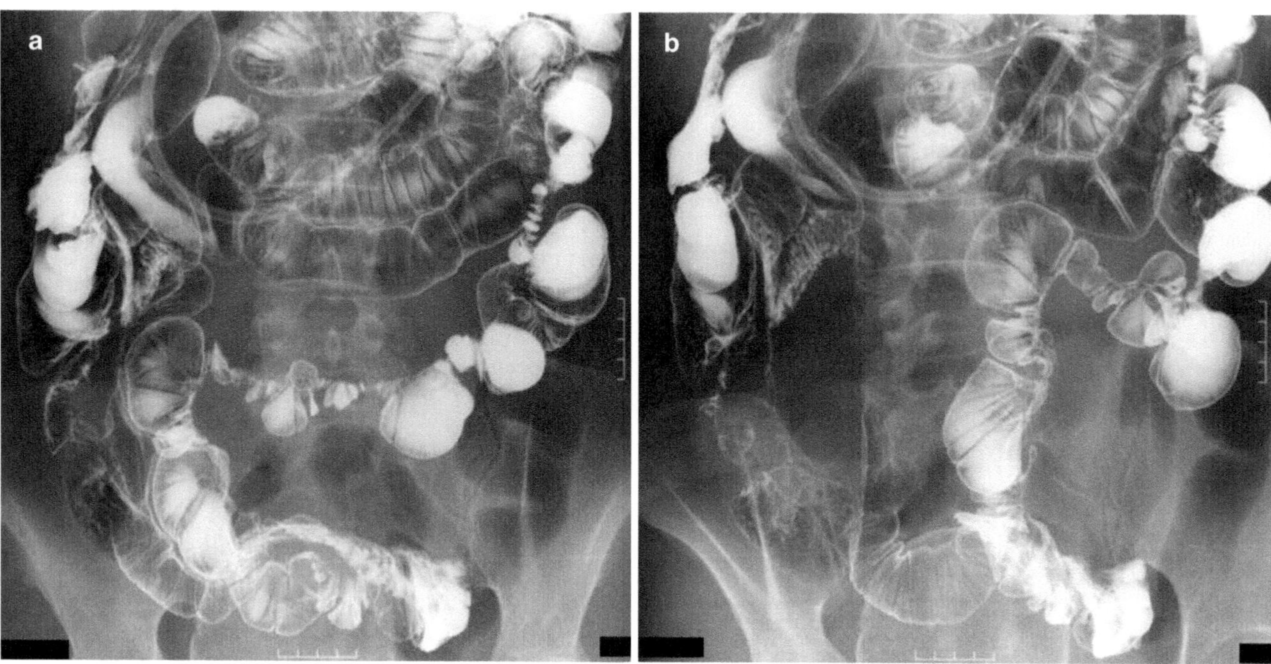

Fig. 13 Double-contrast radiographic image of the small intestine findings: (**a**) Multiple stenoses and longitudinal ulcer in the ileum. (**b**) Stenosis of the ileocolonic anastomosis, but no cancerous lesions were detected grossly, even with contrast, in the resected specimen

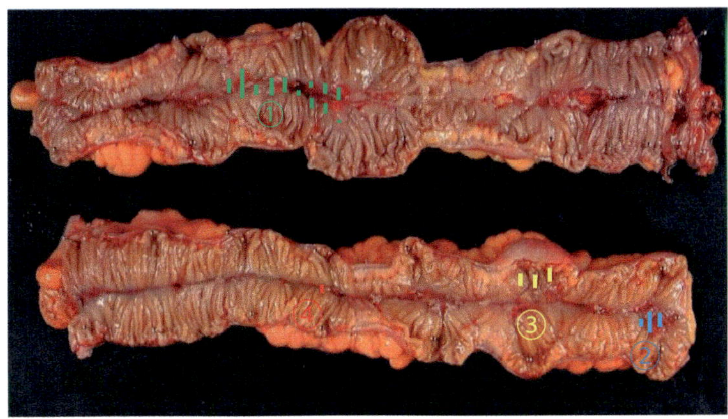

Fig. 14 Gross findings of the resected specimens: The resected specimens show the location of four lesions (①, ②, ③, ④)

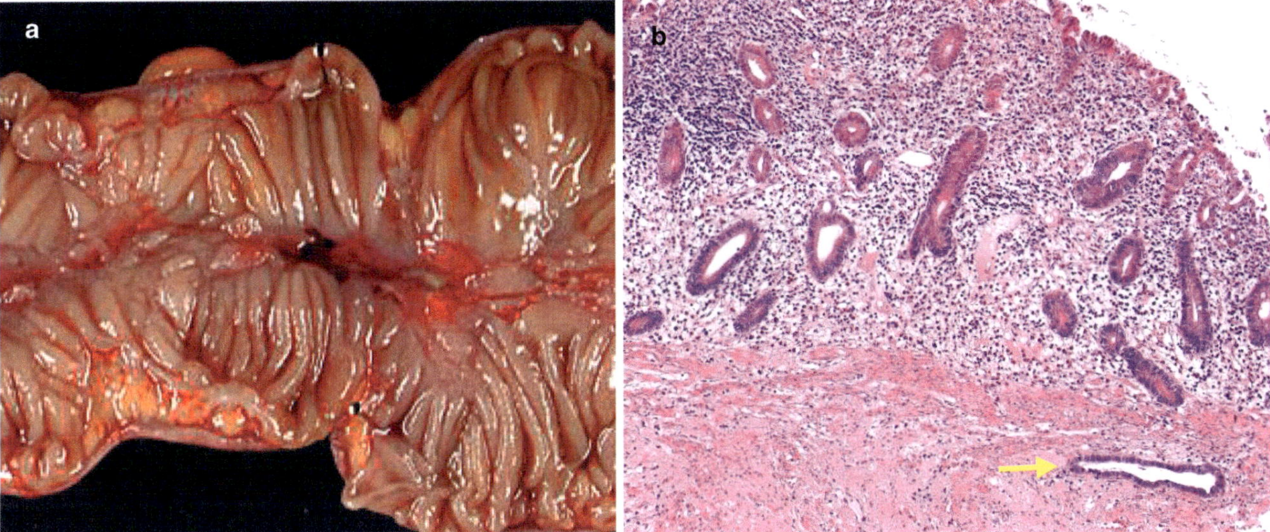

Fig. 15 Close-up view of gross finding and histologic picture of lesion ①: (**a**) The most oral lesion ① was found along with Crohn's ulcer. (**b**) The most oral lesion ① showed mild submucosal invasion (yellow arrow)

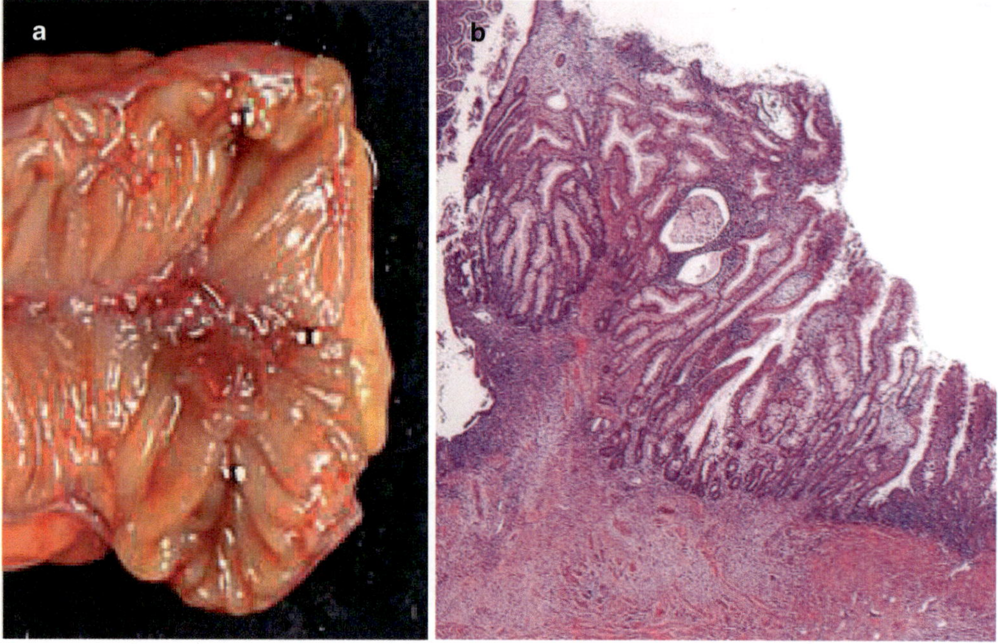

Fig. 16 Close-up view of gross finding and histologic picture of lesion ②. (**a**) Lesion ② was found along with Crohn's ulcer. (**b**) Lesion ② was intramucosal carcinoma

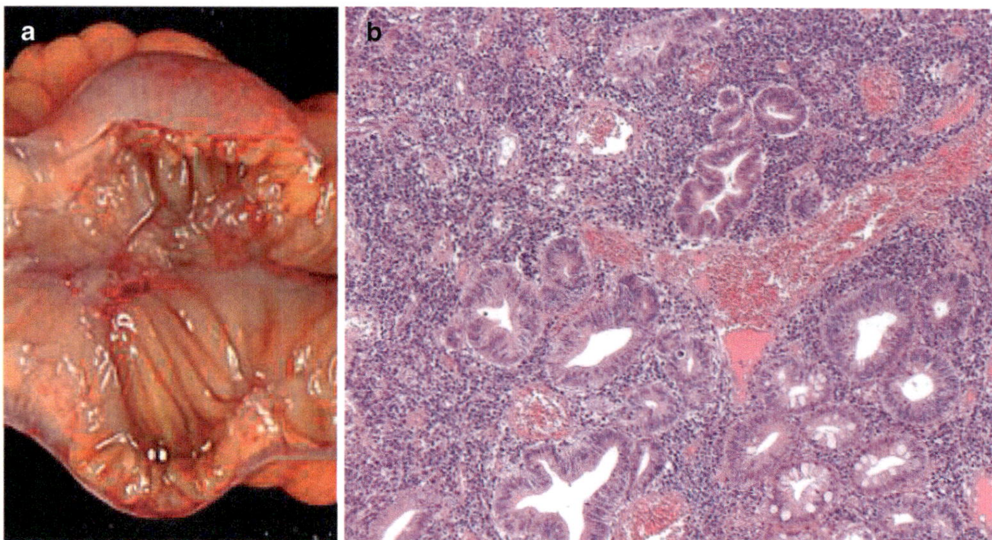

Fig. 17 Close-up view of gross finding and histologic picture of lesion ③. (**a**) Lesion ③ was found near Crohn's ulcer. (**b**) Lesion ③ was intramucosal carcinoma

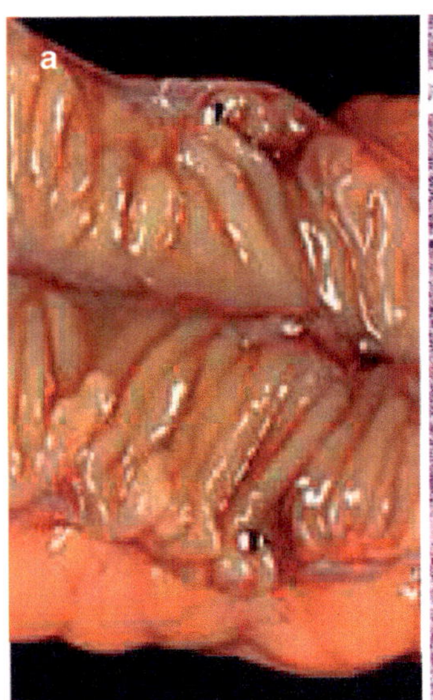

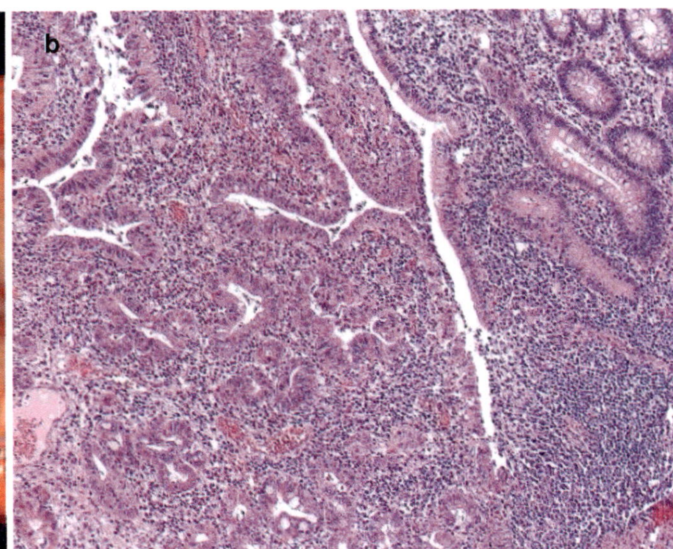

Fig. 18 Close-up view of gross finding and histologic picture of lesion ④. (**a**) Lesion ④ was found along with Crohn's ulcer. (**b**) Lesion ④ was intramucosal carcinoma

The Pathological Diagnosis

- Ileum, all the lesions (①②③④) were not visible grossly
  1. Type 0-IIc, 50 × 15 mm, very well-differentiated adenocarcinoma, pT1a (SM1, 100 μm), Ly0, V0, BD1, pPM0, pDM0, pN0 (lesion ①, green line in Figs. 14, and 15a, b).
  2. Type 0-Is, 10 × 8 mm, well-differentiated adenocarcinoma, pTis, Ly0, V0, BD1, pPM0, pDM0, pN0 (lesion ②, blue line in Figs. 14 and 16a, b).
  3. Type 0-Is, 15 × 10 mm, very well-differentiated adenocarcinoma, pTis, Ly0, V0, BD1, pPM0, pDM0, pN0 (lesion ③, yellow line in Figs. 14 and 17a, b).
  4. Type 0-IIa, 3 × 3 mm, very well-differentiated adenocarcinoma, pTis, Ly0, V0, BD1, pPM0, pDM0, pN0 (lesion ④, red line in Figs. 14 and 18a, b).
- Stage I: pT1a, pN0, M0, P0, H0, R0, Cur A.

Summary

In the present case, a total of four early-stage carcinomas were found near the longitudinal ulcer or at a stenosis of the ileum (Fig. 14) by postoperative pathological examination. The most oral lesion (①) showed mild submucosal invasion (Fig. 15 arrow), and lesions ② to ④ on the anorectal side were all intramucosal carcinomas (Figs. 16, 17, and 18). Early carcinoma arising near a longitudinal ulcer or at a stenosis is clinically difficult to differentiate from ulcer-related changes or inflammatory polyps and is rarely diagnosed preoperatively. In many cases, these lesions can be diagnosed by dividing the resected specimen and carefully examining it.

4 CD Case 4: Advanced Carcinoma of the Ileum with Lateral Growth Tumor-Like Morphology

Keisuke Kawasaki, Koji Ikegami, Minako Fujiwara and Takayuki Matsumoto

40s, female, 10 years of illness

Type of disease: Crohn's disease of the small intestine and colon, Clinical course: Relapsing-remitting

Gross morphology: Superficial elevated type (distinct border)

The patient was diagnosed with Crohn's disease of the small intestine and large intestine type in her 30s, and had been in relapsing-remitting course since then. A radiography (Fig. 19) and a colonoscopy (Fig. 20b–f) performed in 40s revealed a flat elevated lesion in the terminal ileum, which was diagnosed as high-grade dysplasia on biopsy, and ileocecal resection was performed. Histology disclosed advanced carcinoma of the ileum with lateral growth tumor-like morphology (Fig. 21).

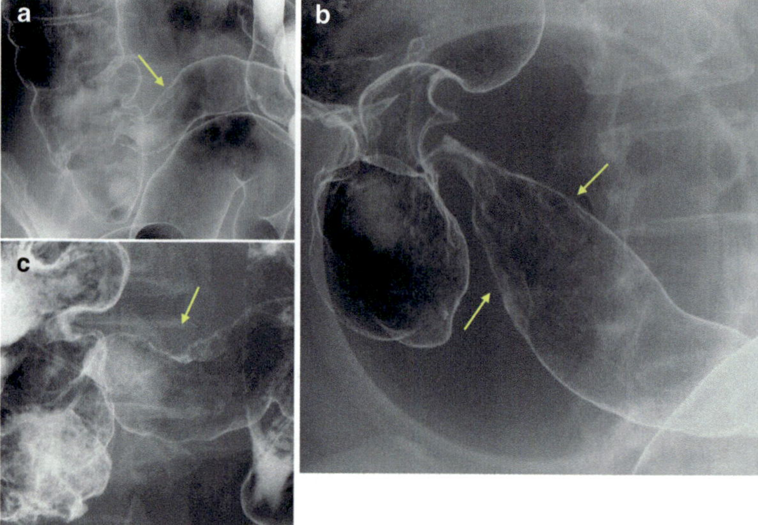

Fig. 19 Double-contrast radiographic findings. (**a**) Terminal ileum, showing raised lesion on mesenteric attachment side (arrow). (**b**) In the frontal view, the lesion is depicted as a flat nodular granular elevated lesion (arrow). (**c**) Lateral deformation was present (arrow)

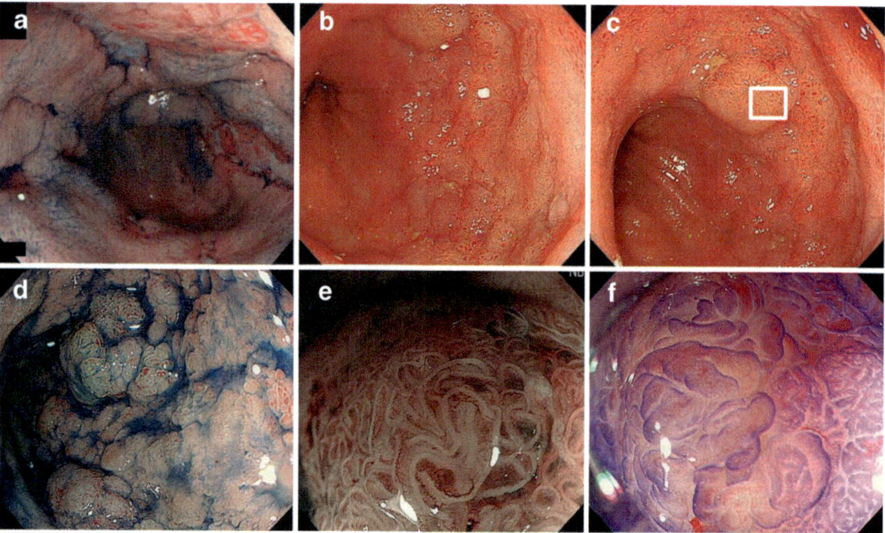

Fig. 20 Lower endoscopic findings. (**a**) Usual observation with chromoendoscopy (8 years ago): longitudinal ulceration in the terminal ileum. (**b**) Normal observation (at the time of operation): the terminal ileum showed a flat granular mucosa with the same color tone as the surrounding mucosa. (**c**) Granules are heterogeneous, with nodules on the oral side. Extension was good. (**d**) Dye-spread image. (**e**) NBI magnified image (white box in **c**). There were few vascular irregularities. (**f**) Magnified image stained with crystal violet (white box in **c**). Dendritic or villous pit was seen. It was considered to be an intramucosal lesion because it was a flat nodular granular elevated lesion in the terminal ileum with lateral deformity on radiography but ulceration in the same area in the past, good extension on conventional endoscopy, and poor vascular and structural irregularity on NBI and dye magnification endoscopy. Surgical resection was performed because the lesion was located in the ileum and was extended more than half circumference

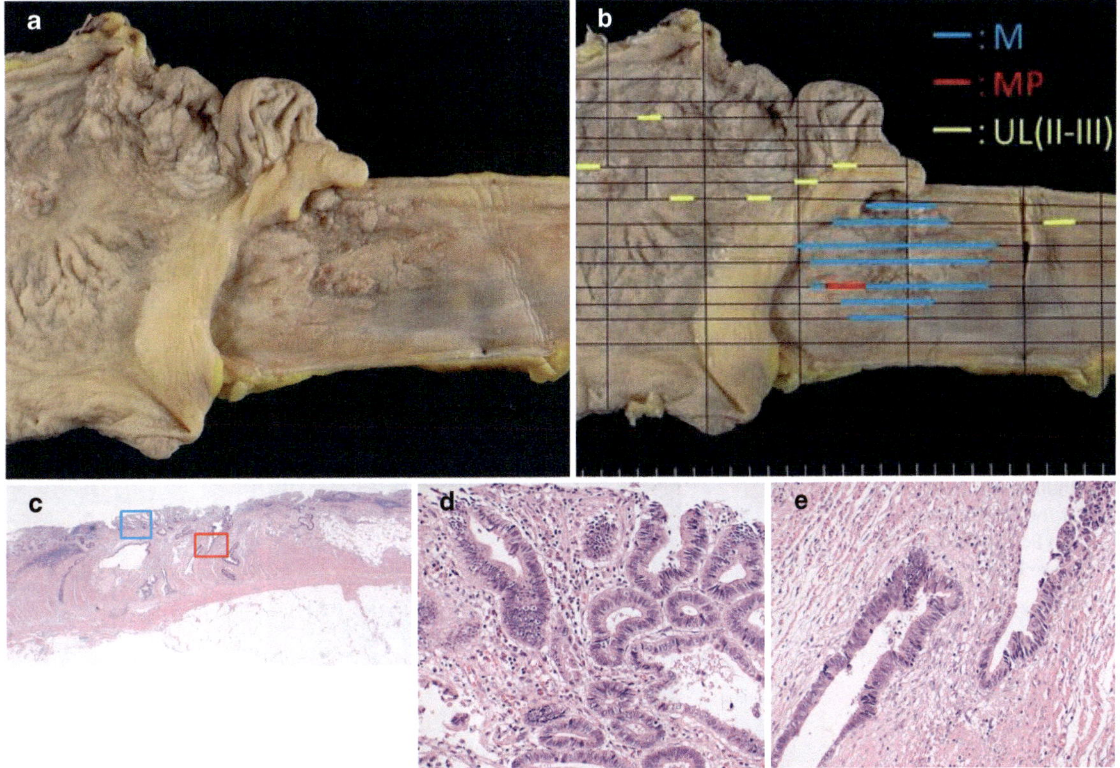

Fig. 21 Histopathological image. (**a**) Resection specimen. A granular, flat, raised lesion was seen in the terminal ileum. (**b**) Mapping, with yellow line for ulcer, blue line for intramucosal carcinoma, and red line for carcinoma invading the muscle layer. (**c**) Loupe image. There was thickening of the muscle layer. (**d**) Magnified image of the blue frame of (**c**) (HE staining). Proliferation of atypical gland ducts corresponding to severe dysplasia was seen in the mucosa. (**e**) Magnified image of the red frame of (**c**) (HE staining). MP infiltration is seen in some areas

Pathological Diagnosis

- Ileum: Type IIa, 53 × 30 mm, well-differentiated adenocarcinoma, pT2 (MP), Ly0, V0, pHM0, pVM0, pN0.
- Stage I: pT2, pN0, M0, P0, H0, R0.

Summary of this Case

A tumor with lateral growth-like morphology arising from a site of active disease 8 years earlier (Fig. 20a). Small and large bowel cancer in CD is reported to occur in highly active lesions, stenoses, and fistulas. Therefore, they are difficult to observe by endoscopy and are often found in advanced cases. In this case, most of the lesions were intramucosal cancer with a distinct border (Fig. 21), and magnified endoscopic observation was possible.

5 Case 5: Ileal Cancer Diagnosed from Left Supraclavicular Fossa Lymph Node Metastasis

Kitaro Futami and Hiroshi Tanabe

40s, female, type S, 29 years of illness

Onset in her teens with diarrhea. One year later, perianal abscess was found. Two years later, she was diagnosed with CD, and treatment was started at our hospital. She underwent bowel resection twice, along with postoperative nutritional management, and immunomodulators and biological agents were introduced at the time of postoperative relapse. Thirteen years after her second surgery, she was hospitalized because of ileus. An enlarged left supraclavicular lymph node was noted at admission (Fig. 22a). Close examinations revealed enlarged lymph nodes at multiple sites (left supraclavicular, paraaortic, and mesenterium) (Fig. 22b). On the radiographic examination of the small intestine, no cancerous lesions were detected (Fig. 23). Based on endoscopy findings (Fig. 24) and a biopsy finding of the left supraclavicular lymph node revealing metastatic adenocarcinoma (Fig. 25), the cancer of the ileum was diagnosed as well- to poorly differentiated adenocarcinoma, which was thought to be the primary lesion (Fig. 26). CEA value: 2.2 ng/mL, CA19-9 value: 292 u/mL.

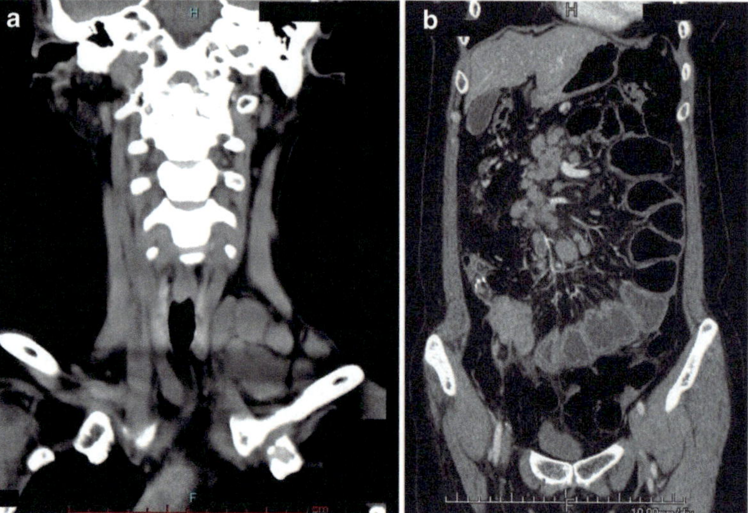

Fig. 22 CT findings: (**a**) Left supraclavicular fossa lymph node enlargement. (**b**) Periaortic, hilar, and mesenteric LN swelling in the abdomen

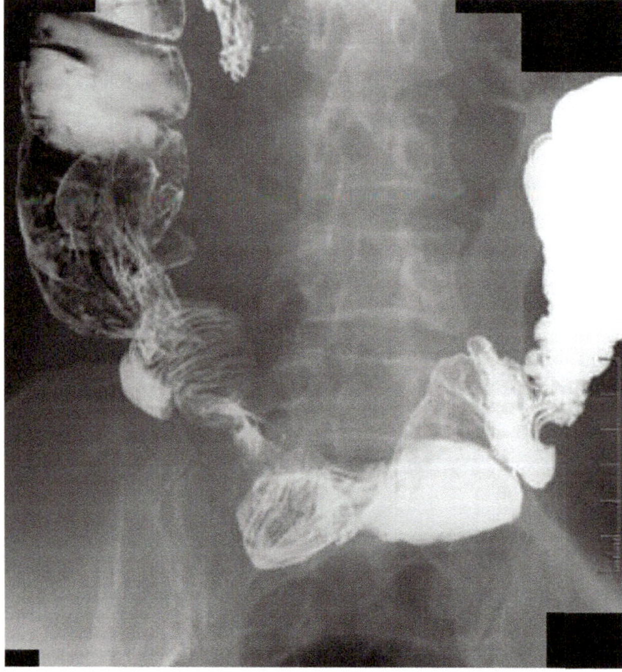

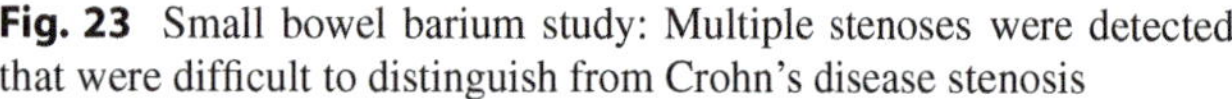

Fig. 23 Small bowel barium study: Multiple stenoses were detected that were difficult to distinguish from Crohn's disease stenosis

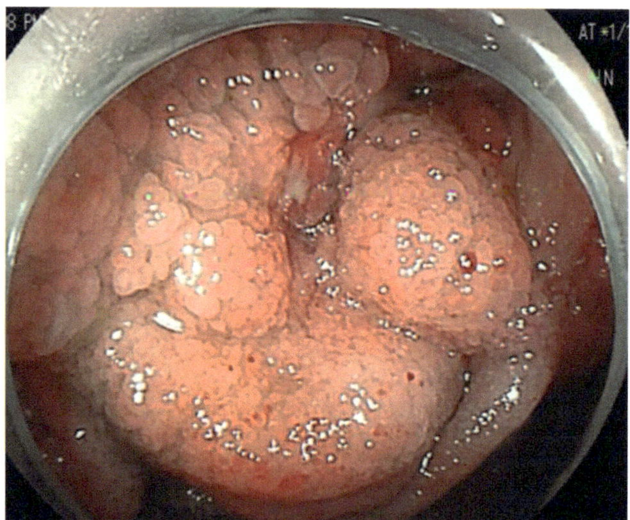

Fig. 24 Small bowel endoscopy: The submucosal tumor-like elevation of the ileal stricture was biopsied, and the pathological findings were determined

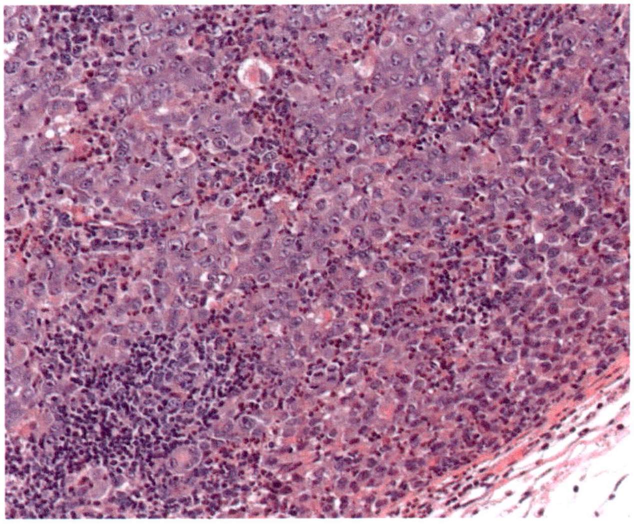

Fig. 25 A biopsy of an enlarged left supraclavicular fossa lymph node: A poorly differentiated adenocarcinoma that was thought to be metastatic

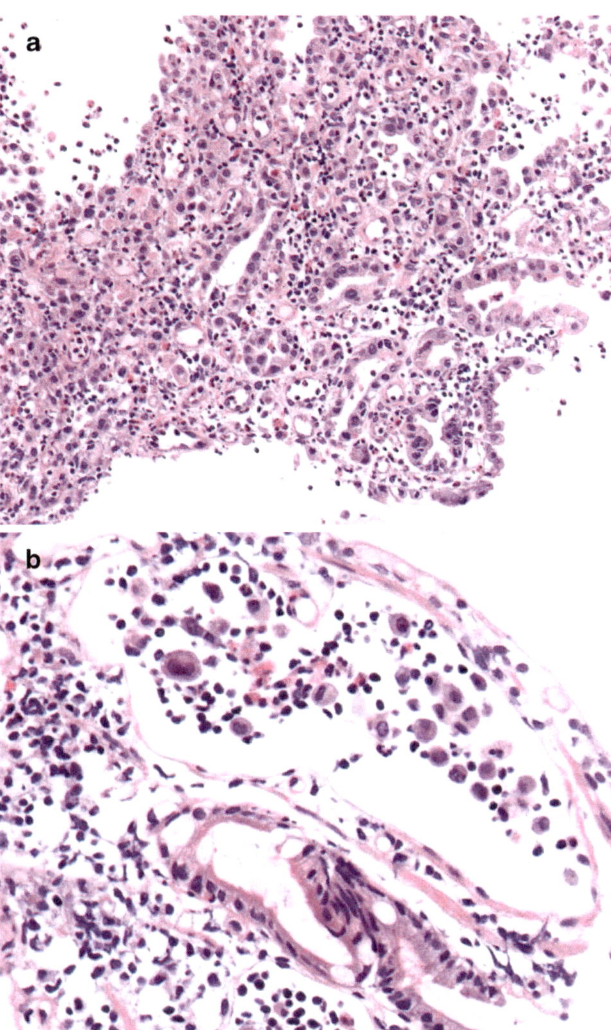

Fig. 26 A biopsy from the ileal stricture: (**a**) A well- to poorly differentiated adenocarcinoma that was thought to be the primary tumor. (**b**) There was invasion of the carcinoma into the dilated lymphatic vessels in the ileal mucosa

The Pathological Diagnosis

- Ileal cancer, circumferential, type 3, well- to poorly differentiated adenocarcinoma,
- Stage IV: M (lymph node) PxH0N4 Tx

Summary

This case was one of ileal cancer diagnosed by left supraclavicular fossa lymph node metastasis. The clinical course and imaging diagnosis of the ileal lesion were difficult.

Colorectal Cancer with Various Features: 15 Cases

Kitaro Futami and Hiroshi Tanabe

K. Futami (✉)
Center for Clinical Medical Research (Surgery), Fukuoka University Chikushi Hospital, Chikushino, Japan

H. Tanabe
Department of Pathology, Fukuoka University Chikushi Hospital, Chikushino, Japan

T. Matsui et al. (eds.), *Atlas of Inflammatory Bowel Disease-Associated Intestinal Cancer*,
https://doi.org/10.1007/978-981-19-3413-1_9

1 Case 6: Carcinoma of the Sigmoid Colon Diagnosed by Preoperative Colonoscopy for Small Bowel Stricture

Kitaro Futami and Hiroshi Tanabe

40s, male, SL type, 22 years of illness

Onset as a teen with perianal lesions. He was diagnosed with CD 2 years later and started treatment. He underwent intestinal surgery twice (small bowel resection and strictureplasty) and multiple anal surgeries with seton drainage. Medical treatment, including biologic agents, was administered for over 20 years, along with home parenteral nutrition. Recently, he began complaining of repeated ileus and underwent surgery because of exacerbation of a small bowel lesion. Preoperative colonoscopy showed a reddish elevated lesion in the sigmoid colon (Fig. 1), and a biopsy revealed well-differentiated adenocarcinoma. CEA value: 1.9 ng/mL, CA19-9 value: 5.0 u/mL.

Surgery

1. Sigmoidectomy and lymph node dissection end-to-end anastomosis.
2. Partial resection of the ileum with side-to-side anastomosis for Crohn's disease.

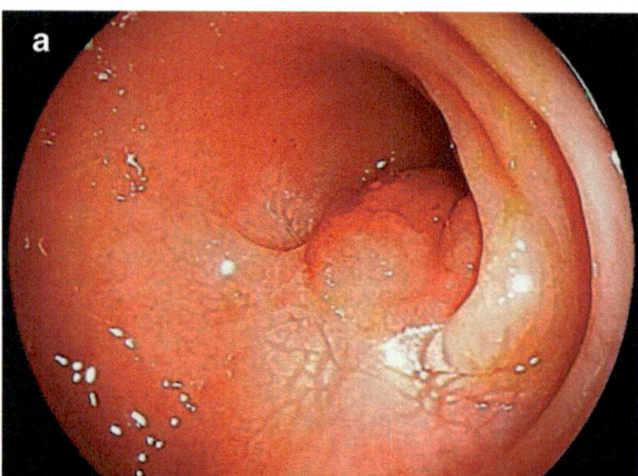

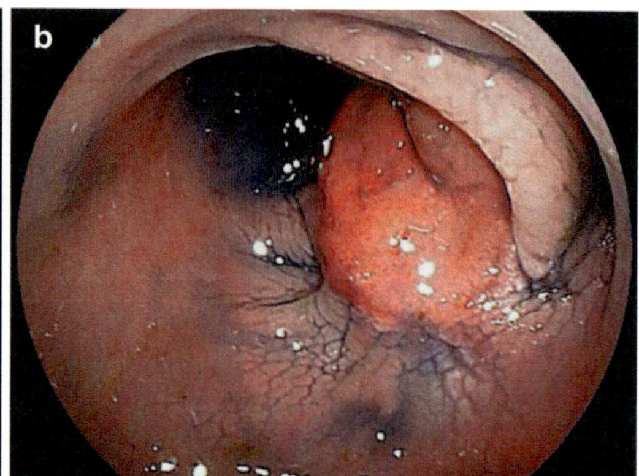

Fig. 1 Endoscopic findings: (**a**) Reddish elevated lesion (30 mm in diameter). (**b**) Chromoendoscopic view revealing converging folds

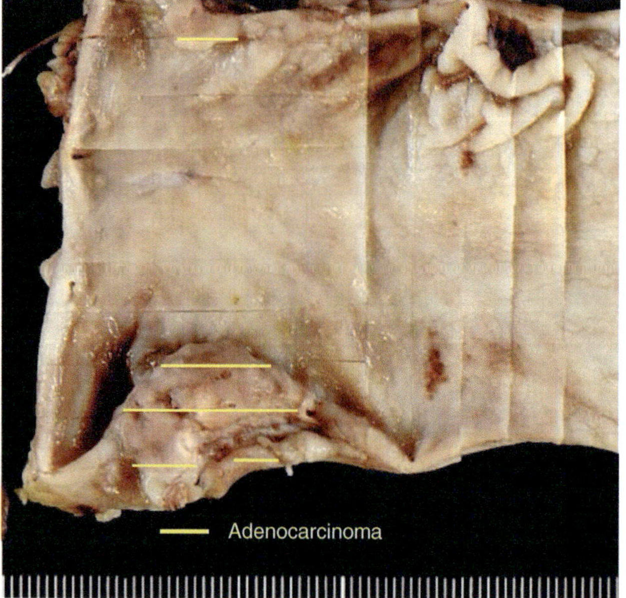

Fig. 2 Gross finding of the resected specimen: Is-like elevated lesion of 20 mm in length was found in the sigmoid colon (yellow line)

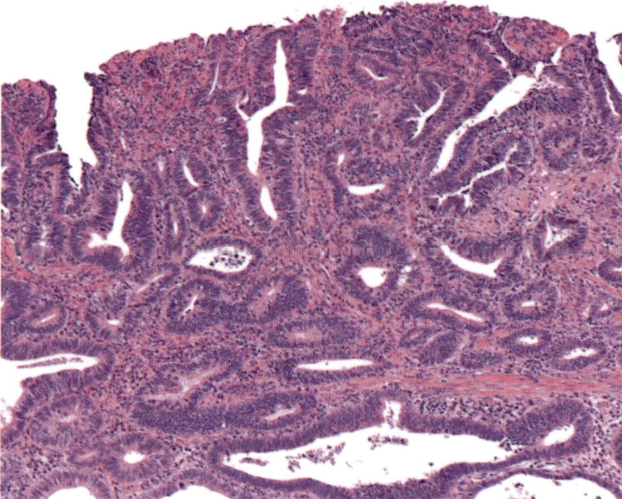

Fig. 3 H.E. staining: Well-differentiated tubular adenocarcinoma. There was no obvious adenomatous component within the tumor

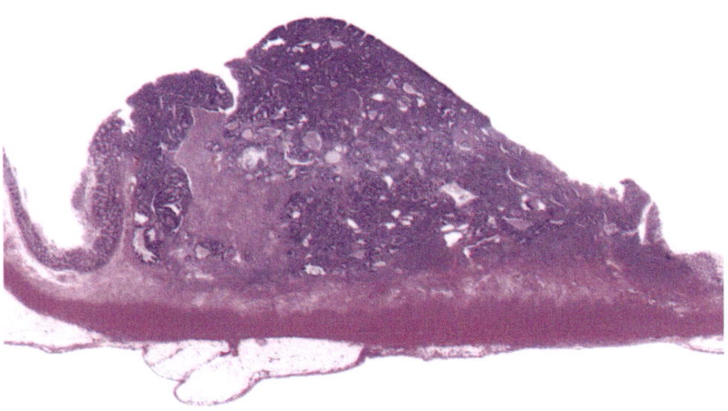

Fig. 4 Loupe view of the tumor: The carcinoma had invaded deep into the sigmoid colon wall

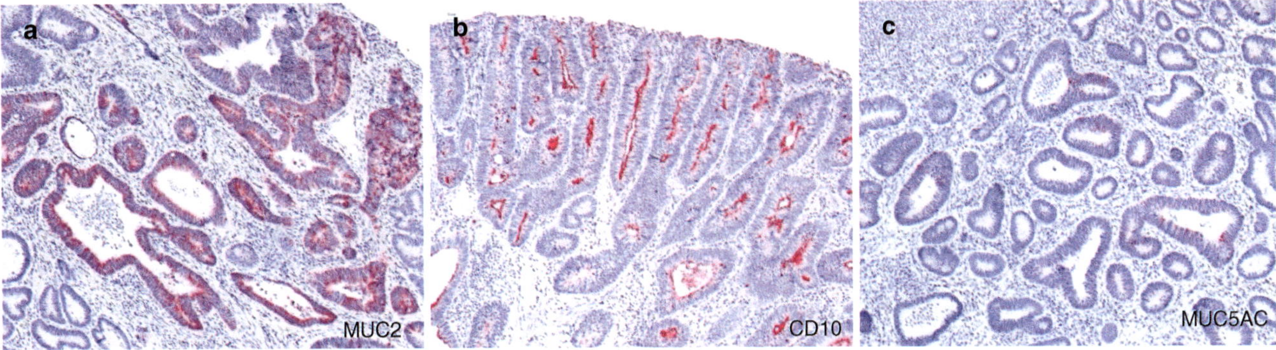

Fig. 5 Immunohistochemical staining: (**a** and **b**) Most of the tumor cells were positive for MUC2 (**a**) and CD-10 (**b**) with a predominance of intestinal-type mucin phenotype. (**c**) A small number were positive for MUC5AC, and some showed gastric-type mucin phenotype

The Pathological Diagnosis

- Sigmoid colon: Type 0-Is, 20 × 15 mm, well-differentiated adenocarcinoma, pT1b (SM, 7500 μm), Ly0, V0, INF b, BD1, pPM0, pDM0, pN0.
- Stage I: pT1b, pN0, M0, P0, H0, R0, Cur A.

Summary

Well-differentiated tubular adenocarcinoma had invaded deep into the sigmoid colon wall (Figs. 2, 3, and 4). There was no obvious adenomatous component within the tumor. The tumor mucin phenotype was a mixed gastric and intestinal mucin phenotype (Fig. 5). The lack of an adenomatous component in the lesion and the mixed gastrointestinal trait suggested that this was an inflammatory bowel disease-associated carcinoma. Since the pathway of inflammatory bowel disease-associated carcinoma is usually different from that of colorectal carcinoma, the absence of an adenoma component is not uncommon.

2 Case 7: Ascending Colon Cancer Diagnosed by Scrutiny Endoscopy for Recurrent Abdominal Pain

Kitaro Futami and Hiroshi Tanabe

50s, female, type L, 24.8 years of illness

Onset in her 20s with bloody stool. However, for 11 years, she did not undergo any medical treatment. In her 40s, she developed perianal abscess, which was diagnosed as CD and treated with drainage. Medical treatment with biologics was started at that point. After 2 years, colonoscopy revealed erosions at the ascending colon and inflammatory polyps, in which a biopsy showed no cancerous tissue. Three years later, she complained of right lower quadrant pain and increased frequency of defecation. Colonoscopy showed a circumferential type 2 lesion in the ascending colon (Fig. 6), and a biopsy showed poorly differentiated adenocarcinoma with signet ring cells. Barium radiography showed apple core finding in the ascending colon (Fig. 7). CEA value: 3.6 ng/mL, CA19-9 value: 17.0 u/mL.

Surgery

Right hemicolectomy, lymph node dissection, end-to-end anastomosis

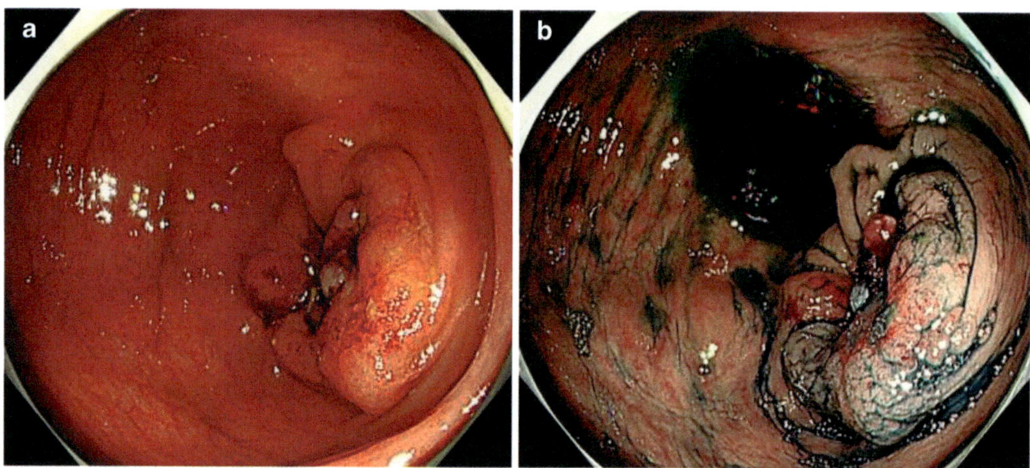

Fig. 6 Endoscopic findings: (**a**) A total circumferential type 2 lesion was found in the ascending colon. (**b**) Chromoendoscopic view revealing fine granularity

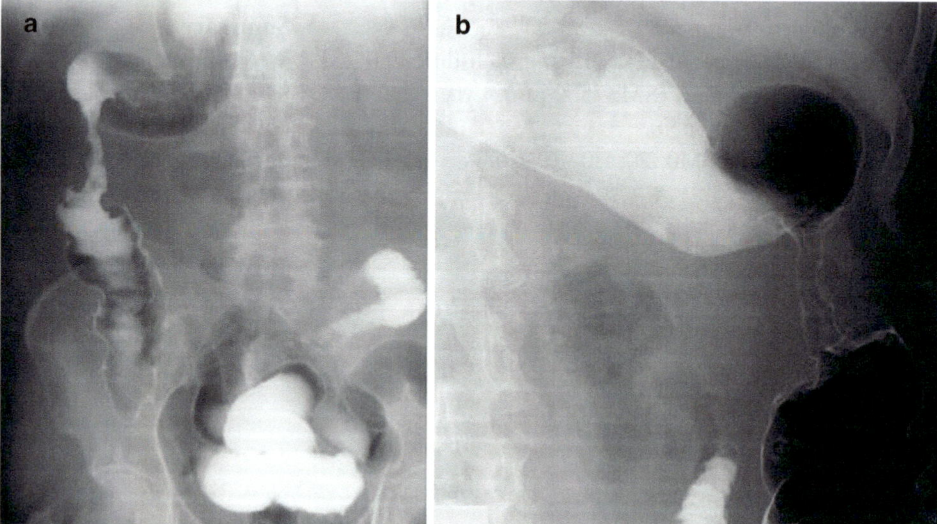

Fig. 7 Barium radiographic findings: Supine position (**a**): Apple core findings were noted in the ascending colon. Prone position (**b**): A long and severe stricture. of the ascending colon

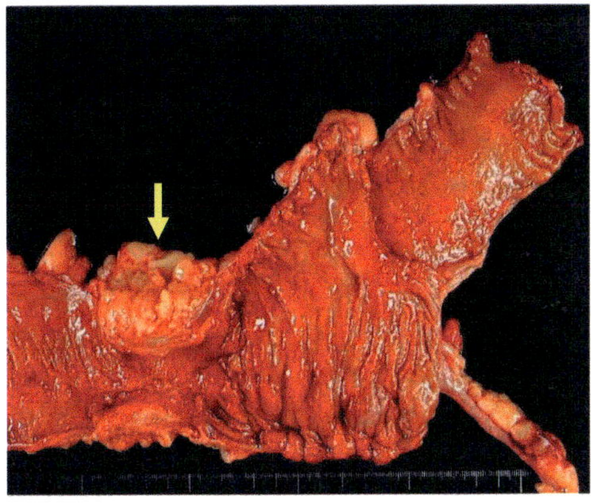

Fig. 8 Gross finding of the resected specimen: The total circumferential type 3 tumor of the ascending colon (yellow arrow) caused slight dilatation of the oral bowel, and the mucosa was edematous

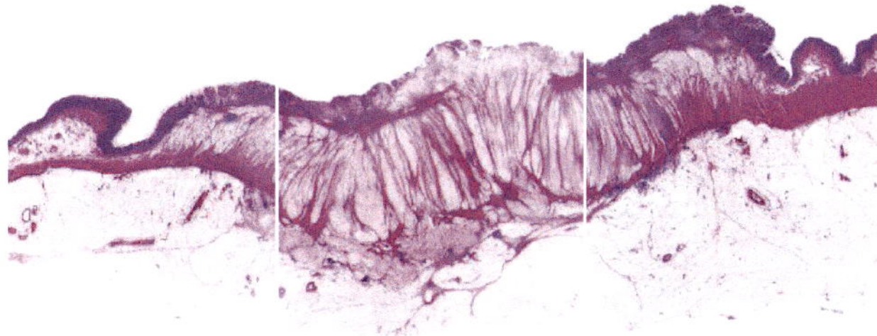

Fig. 9 Loupe view of the tumor: The tumor was a mucinous carcinoma that had invaded the whole thickness

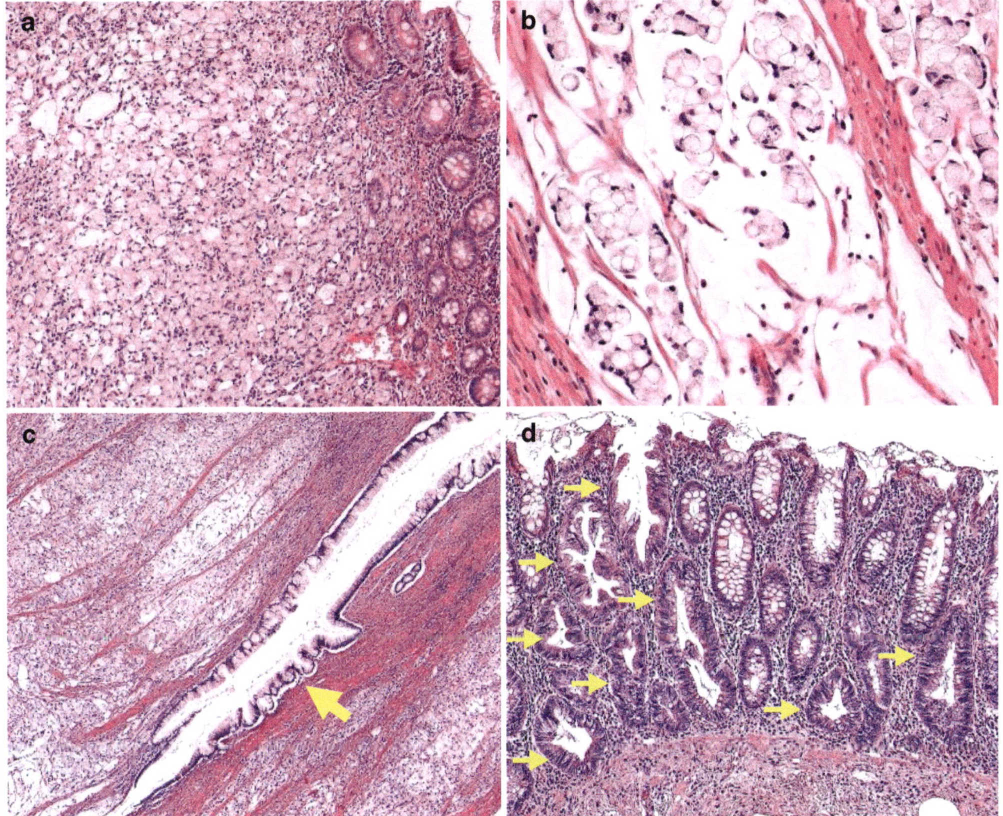

Fig. 10 Microscopic findings of the tumor: (**a**) Most of the carcinoma cells showed intracellular mucous degeneration. (**b**) Cancer cells suspended in extracellular mucous degeneration showed cellular adhesion. (**c**) Very well-differentiated adenocarcinoma (arrow) was also observed. (**d**) In addition, a small dysplastic epithelium was found near the anal part of the lesion (arrows)

The Pathological Diagnosis

- Ascending colon: Type 3, 70 mm, very well- to poorly differentiated adenocarcinoma with marked intra- and extracellular mucous degeneration (mucinous adenocarcinoma) (Figs. 8 and 9) and dysplastic epithelium (Fig. 10d), pT4a (SE), Ly1b, V1a, INF b, Pn1a, pPM0, pDM0, pN2a.
- Stage IIIc: pT4a, pN2a, M0, P0, H0, R0, Cur A.

Summary

The total circumferential type 3 tumor of the ascending colon (Fig. 8 yellow arrow). Pathologically, the tumor was a mucinous adenocarcinoma that had invaded the whole thickness (Fig. 9). Most of the carcinoma cells showed intracellular mucinous degeneration (Fig. 10a) and very well-differentiated adenocarcinoma (arrow in Fig. 10c) was also observed. Inflammatory bowel disease-associated carcinoma has a high frequency of mucinous adenocarcinoma, and there are many lesions with a variety of histological features (Fig. 10).

3 Case 8: Intraoperatively Confirmed Transverse Colon Cancer of the Scirrhous Type

Kitaro Futami and Hiroshi Tanabe

20s, male, SL type, 2 years of illness

Onset in his 20s with perianal fistula. One year after the onset, he complained of abdominal pain and was diagnosed with SL type CD after a close examination. A stenotic lesion 10 cm long with wall thickening in the splenic flexure of the transverse colon was detected by CT as well as by a barium study (Figs. 11 and 12). Colonoscopy showed circumferential stenosis at the splenic flexure (Fig. 13), with negative biopsy results. A biopsy of a rectal erosion revealed granuloma. Small bowel radiography found ulcers with deformity in the pelvic ileum. Perianal lesions showed multiple fistula scars and skin tags. CEA value: 1.6 ng/mL, CA19-9 value: 23 u/mL.

Surgery

Left-sided resection of the transverse colon, lymph node dissection, end-to-end anastomosis. An intraoperative rapid pathological examination detected mucinous adenocarcinoma.

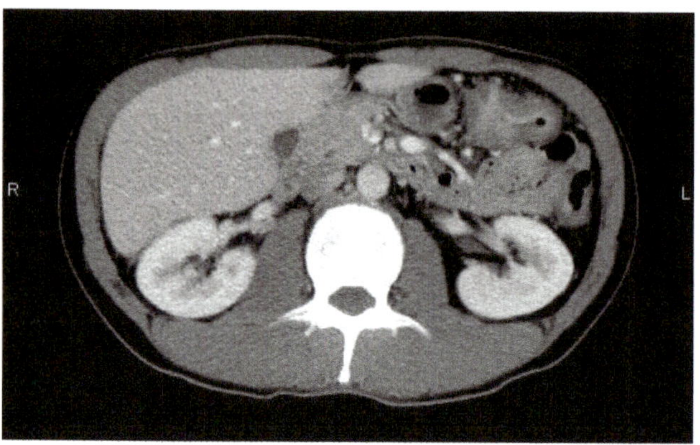

Fig. 11 CT findings: Stenotic lesion with wall thickening in the transverse colon at the splenic flexure

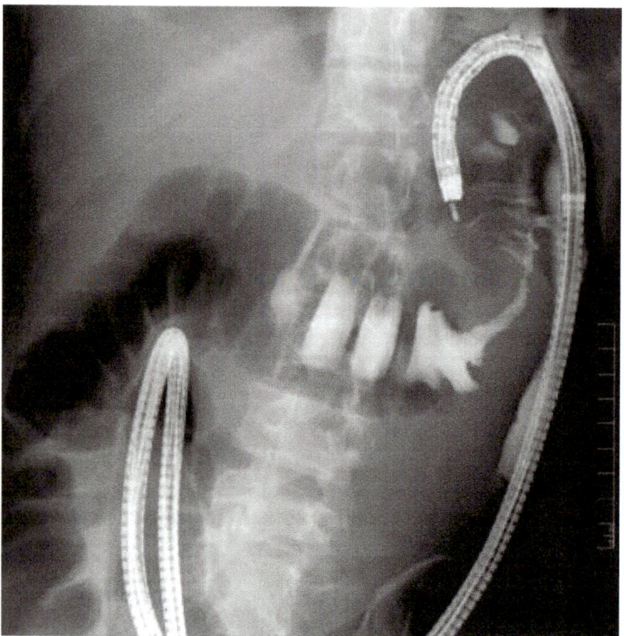

Fig. 12 Barium enema findings: Radiographic depiction of the circumferential stenosis of the splenic flexure using soluble contrast media through colonoscope

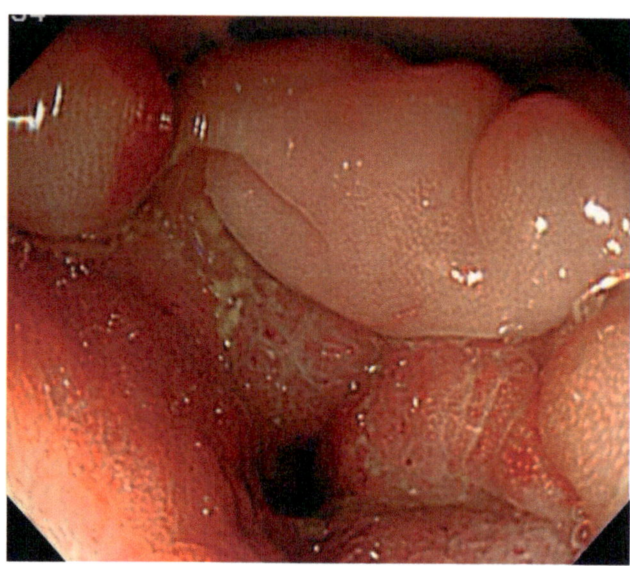

Fig. 13 Colonoscopy findings: Stenosis of the transverse colon, which was speculated to be a tumor, was noted, but a biopsy did not show any cancer cells

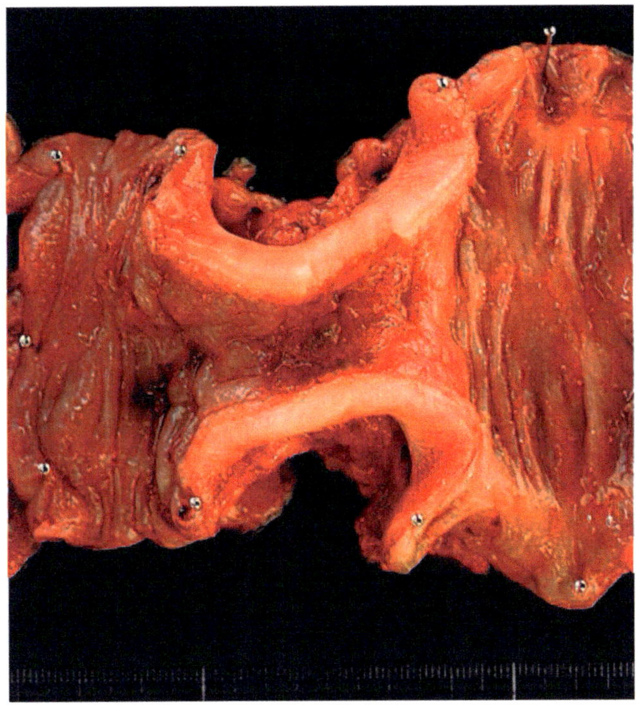

Fig. 14 Gross finding of the resected specimen: The lumen was narrowed due to a circumferential type 3 advanced carcinoma of the transverse colon, and the oral intestine was slightly dilated

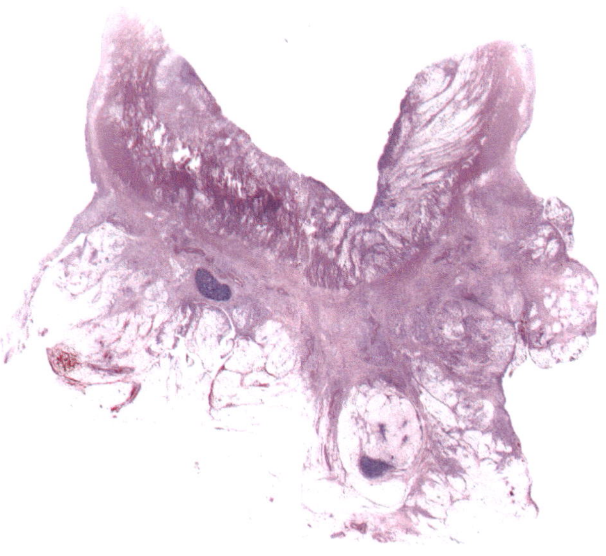

Fig. 15 Loupe findings: The tumor was type 3 advanced carcinoma of the transverse colon

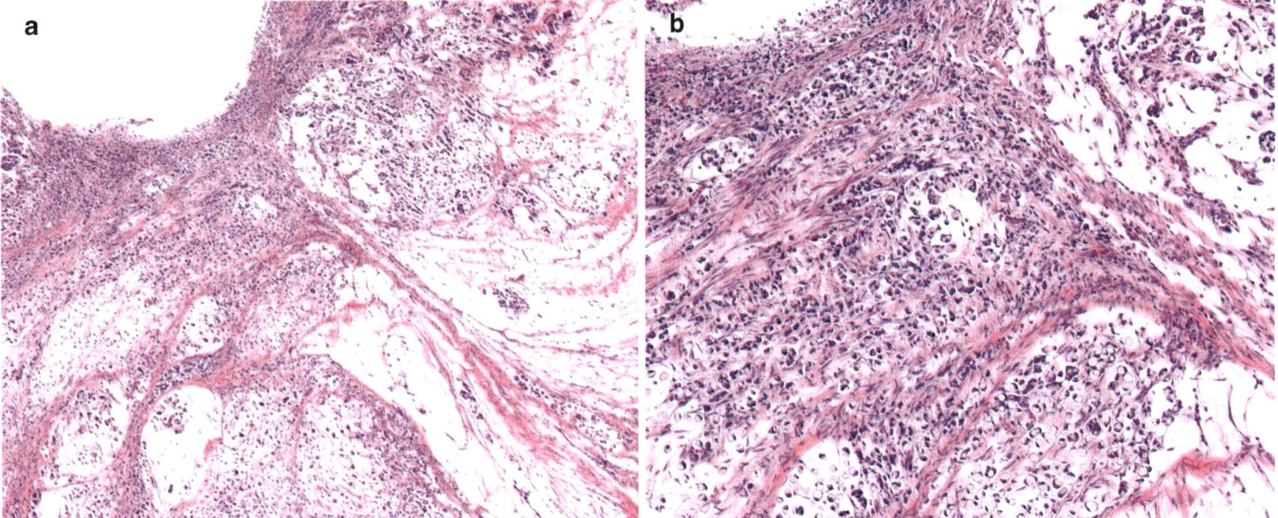

Fig. 16 H.E. staining: (**a**) The lesion was a mucinous adenocarcinoma caused by poorly differentiated adenocarcinoma with marked vascular invasion. (**b**) Close-up view of (**a**)

The Pathological Diagnosis

- Transverse colon: Type 3, 50 mm, poorly differentiated adenocarcinoma with marked intra- and extracellular mucous degeneration (mucinous adenocarcinoma, pT4a (SE), Ly1c, V1b, INF c, Pn1b, pPM0, pDM0, pN2b.
- Stage IIIc: pT4a, pN2b, M0, P0, H0, R0, Cur A.

Summary

The tumor was type 3 advanced carcinoma of the transverse colon and was pathologically mucinous adenocarcinoma with marked vascular invasion (Figs. 14, 15, and 16) and multiple lymph node metastases. Most of the colorectal cancers associated with Crohn's disease in Japan occur in the rectosigmoid region, and other sites are rare, as in Case 7. However, mucinous adenocarcinoma is the most common histological type, as well as carcinoma arising in the rectum and anus.

4 Case 9: Upper Rectal Cancer Diagnosed by Multiple Biopsies

Kitaro Futami and Hiroshi Tanabe

30s, male, SL type, 19 years of illness

Onset in his teens with a perianal fistula. At the same time, CD was diagnosed and nutritional therapy started. Five years later, the perianal fistula recurred, and seton drainage was successfully performed. Ten years later, ileocecal-rectal fistula was found and followed conservatively. Eighteen years after the onset of the disease, he complained of obstructive symptoms, ileorectal fistula, anal stenosis, extensive perianal fistula, and abscess.

First, an anal procedure (incision, seton method, and biopsy) was performed under anesthesia, followed by bowel surgery (bowel resection, ileostomy, and upper rectal wedge resection). Eight months after the operation, endoscopy was performed for follow-up, and edematous erythematous mucosa was observed in the narrowed part of the upper rectum. Three biopsies were performed before the final diagnosis of mucinous adenocarcinoma was obtained (Fig. 17a–c). Computed tomography revealed no localized lesion or metastatic findings, and barium contrast radiography revealed skipped ulcer scars throughout the colon, transverse and descending colonic stenosis over 4 cm of the upper rectum. CEA value: 2.3 ng/mL, CA19-9 value: 1.0 u/mL.

Surgery

Total proctocolectomy (rectal amputation), lymph node dissection, ileostomy

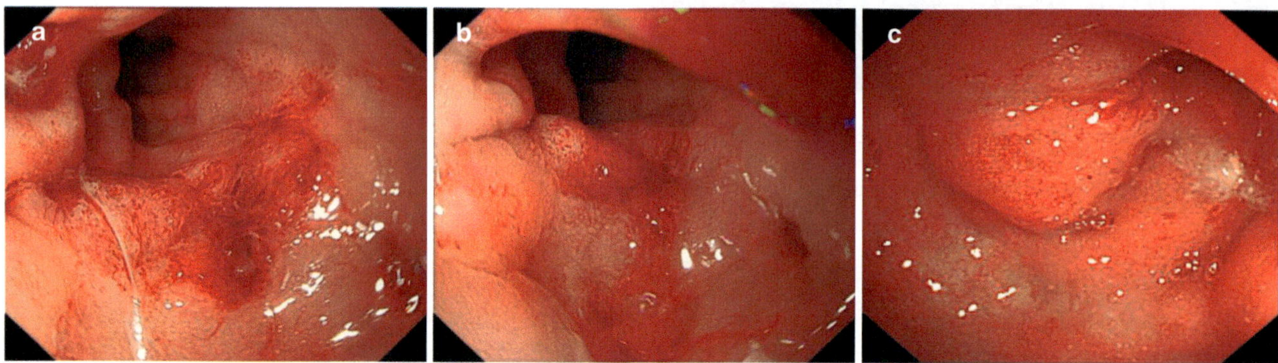

Fig. 17 Colonoscopy: (**a**) Reddish edematous mucosa in the upper rectal stenosis. (**b**) Easy bleeding mucosa with unevenness. (**c**) A submucosal tumor-like elevation on the anorectal side were noted

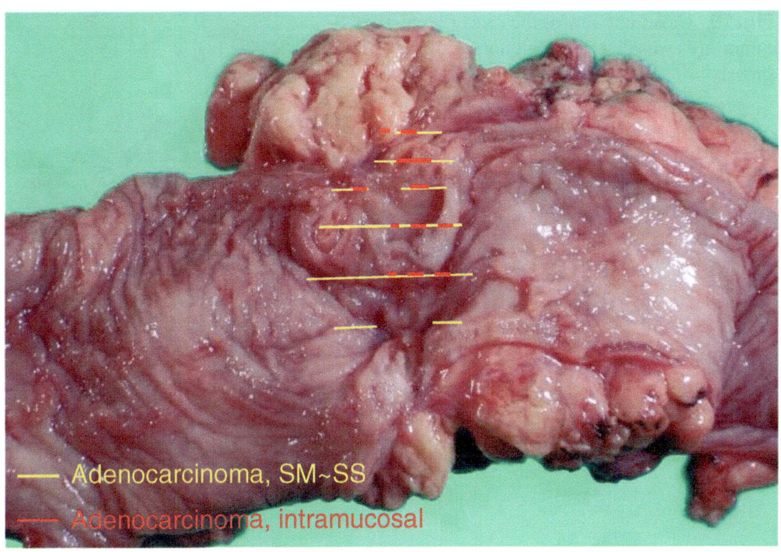

Fig. 18 Macroscopic finding of the resected rectum: An almost circumferential stenosing tumor with intestinal distention in the rectum (Ra). Intramucosal cancer area was presented in red line cancer. Cancer invasion areas down to the submucosa and subserosa were shown in yellow line. The mucosa consisted of small nests of very well-differentiated tubular adenocarcinoma interspersed with non-neoplastic inflammatory polyps, which made it difficult to recognize the lesions macroscopically

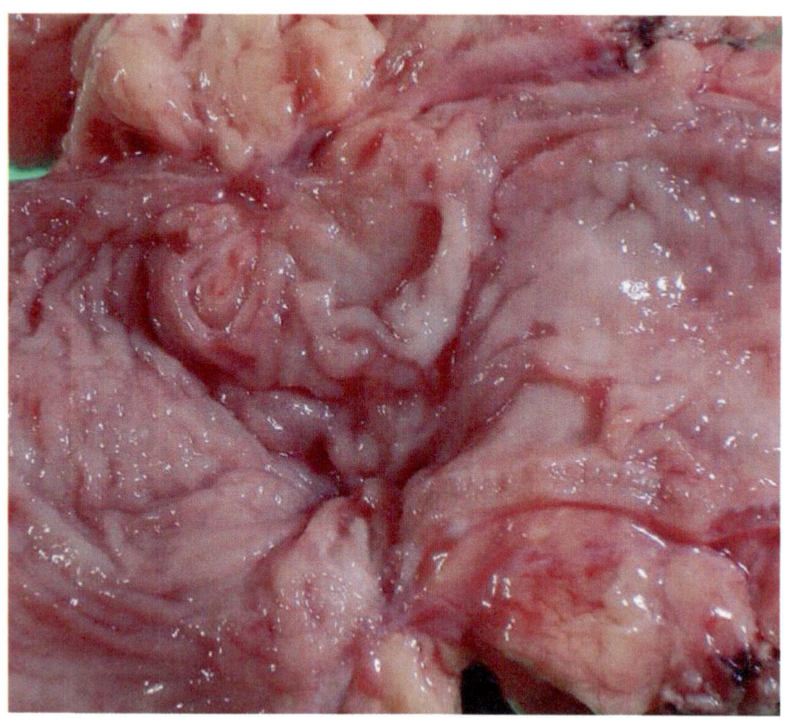

Fig. 19 Close-up view of the cancer area: The tumor area was deformed but not identified grossly

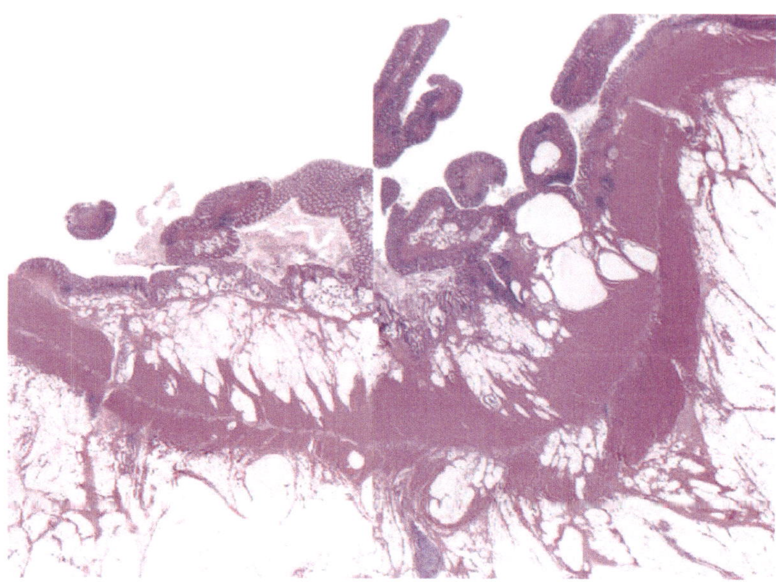

Fig. 20 Loupe finding of the tumor: The carcinoma invaded all layers but there was a lack of fibrotic stromal reaction in the cancer-invaded area with strong mucous degeneration, and there were non-neoplastic inflammatory polyps on the inner surface of the tumor

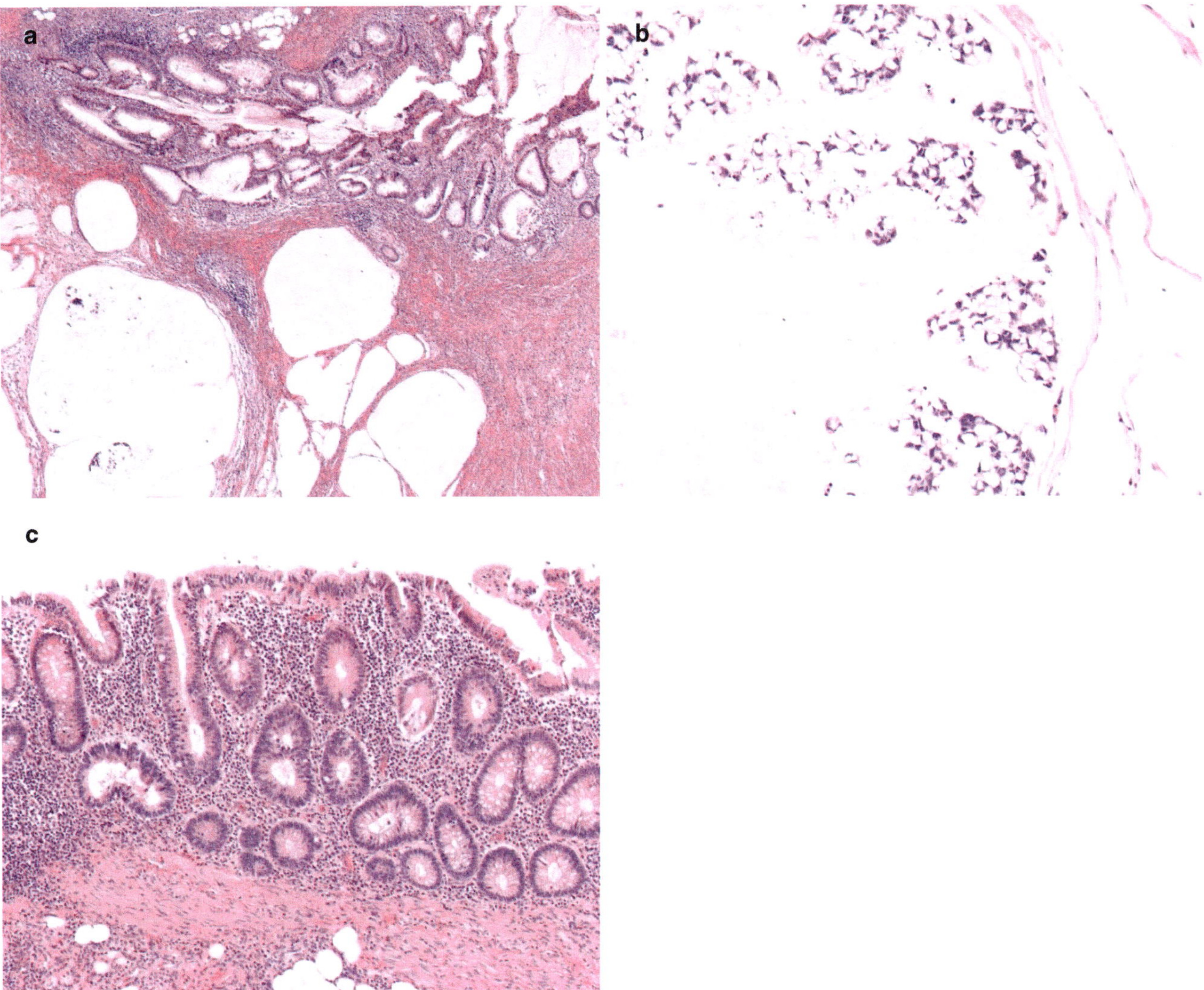

Fig. 21 H.E. staining: (**a** and **b**) An advanced carcinoma that mainly comprised very well-differentiated tubular adenocarcinoma with intra- and extracellular mucous degeneration. (**c**) In the surrounding area, scattered foci of dysplastic epithelium were found

The Pathological Diagnosis

- Rectum: Type 5, 40 mm, very well- to well-differentiated adenocarcinoma with intra- and extracellular mucous degeneration and dysplastic epithelium, pT3 (SS), Ly0, V0, BD1, INF b, Pn1a, pPM0 pDM0, pN0.
- Stage IIa: pT3, pN0, M0, P0, H0, R0, Cur A

Summary

Pathologically, this tumor was difficult to identify grossly (Figs. 18 and 19), because the mucosa consisted of small nests of very well-differentiated tubular adenocarcinoma interspersed with non-neoplastic inflammatory polyps (Figs. 20 and 21). In addition, there was a lack of fibrotic stromal reaction in the cancer-invaded area with strong mucous degeneration and fibrosis in the surrounding non-neoplastic submucosa. The fibrosis in the surrounding non-tumor submucosa may have been induced by the inflammation due to Crohn's disease or the effect of a previous wedge resection procedure. Inflammatory bowel disease-associated cancers are often difficult to recognize or have an atypical gross appearance. This may be due to background factors such as inflammation, ulceration and scarring, fistulas, and the presence of inflammatory polyps, as well as the nature of the tumor itself, including its degree of differentiation, presentation, mode of invasion, and extracellular mucus degeneration. In the present case, the mucosal lesion showed faint color changes and was difficult to diagnose colonoscopically. In addition, the biopsy site was questionable, and repeated biopsies were necessary before a definite cancer diagnosis was obtained.

5 Case 10: Lower Rectal and Anal Cancer with Extensive Perianal Invasion Diagnosed by an Outpatient Biopsy

Kitaro Futami and Hiroshi Tanabe

30s, female, SL type, 12.5 years of illness

Onset in her 20s with abdominal symptoms. The diagnosis was made and she underwent anorectal surgery in the same year. Five years later, bowel surgery (two resection procedures) was performed, and anal dilation continued. She was diagnosed with exacerbation of an anorectal lesion and received treatment for 7 months, but her condition did not improve, so she was referred to our hospital. At the same time, the cancer was diagnosed by a transanal biopsy (Fig. 22). The cancer was diagnosed as a circular anorectal lesion with invading adjacent organs on close examinations (Figs. 23, 24, and 25). CEA value: 17.0 ng/mL, CA19-9 value: 57.0 u/mL.

Surgery

Posterior total pelvic exenteration, lymph node dissection, sigmoid colostomy

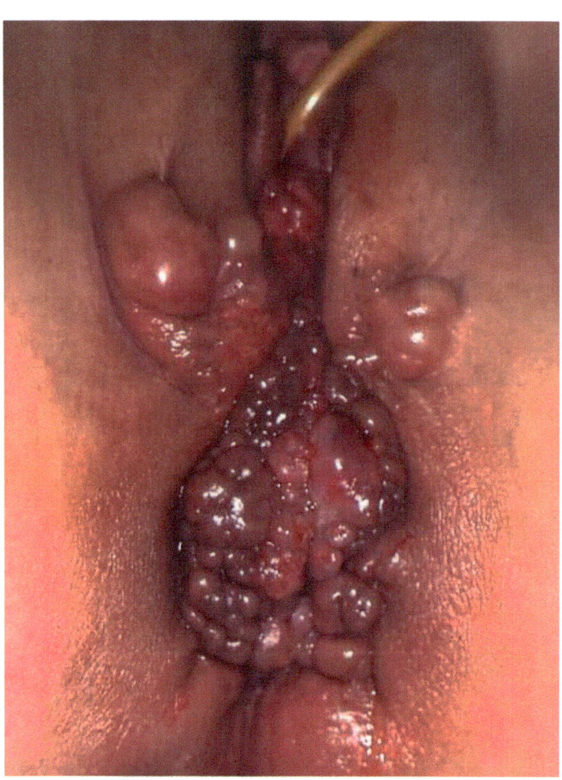

Fig. 22 Perianal findings: Circular anal sclerosis, mass at the site of previous fistula, mass formation in the vagina. An ambulatory biopsy performed under anesthesia showed cancer tissue

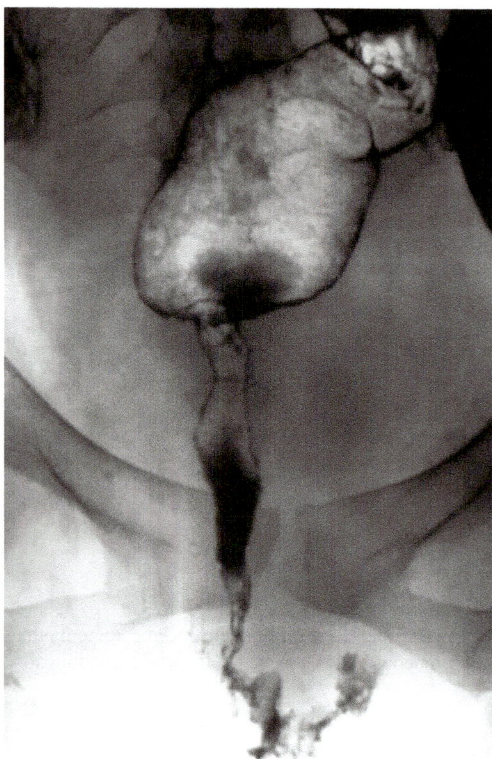

Fig. 23 Barium enema findings: Stenotic lesion from the lower rectum to the anus, 11 cm long

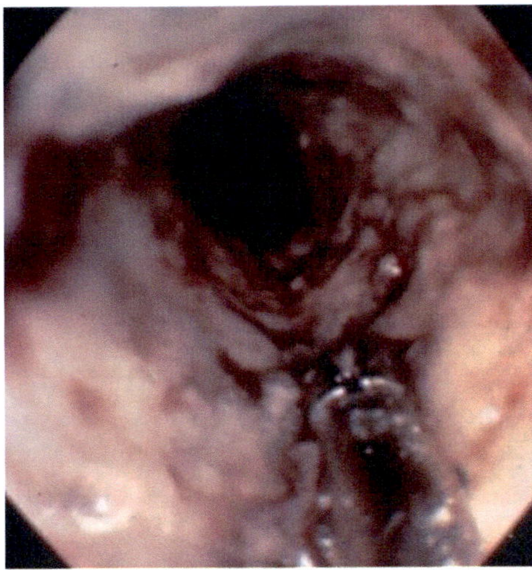

Fig. 24 Endoscopic findings: Rectal and anal stenosis and irregular ulceration with uneven granularity

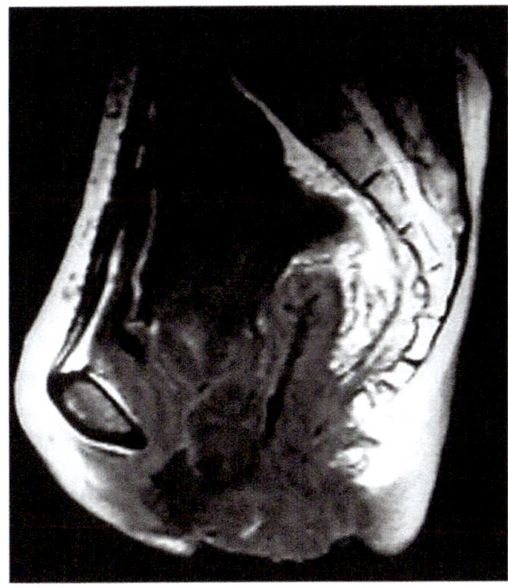

Fig. 25 MRI findings: The wall thickness suggested tumor invasion of the lower rectum to perineal region

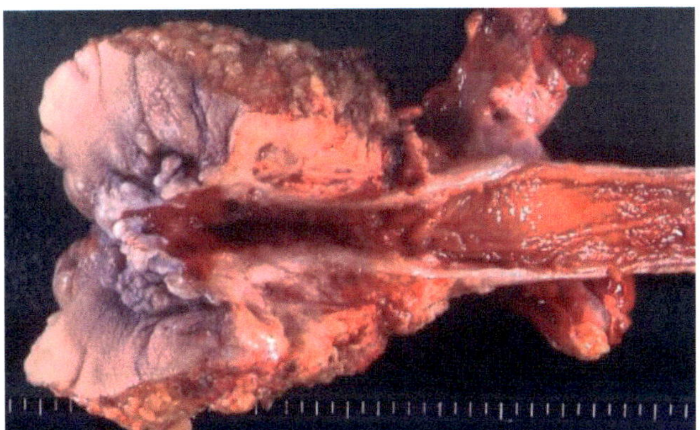

Fig. 26 Gross findings: Cancer of the lower rectum and anus type 3, total circumference, tumor invasion of the uterus and vagina

The Pathological Diagnosis

- Rectum and anal canal: Type 3, 90 mm, mucous adenocarcinoma with signet ring cell carcinoma, pT4b (vagina, uterus), Ly1c, V1b, pPM0, pDM0, pRM0.
- Stage IIIc: pT4b, pN3, M0, P0, H0, R0, Cur A.

Summary

Postoperative pathological examination revealed that the rectal and anal canal tumor was a type 3 cancer (Fig. 26) and histologically it was mucinous adenocarcinoma (Fig. 27).

This case was diagnosed based on visual findings and palpation of the anal region alone.

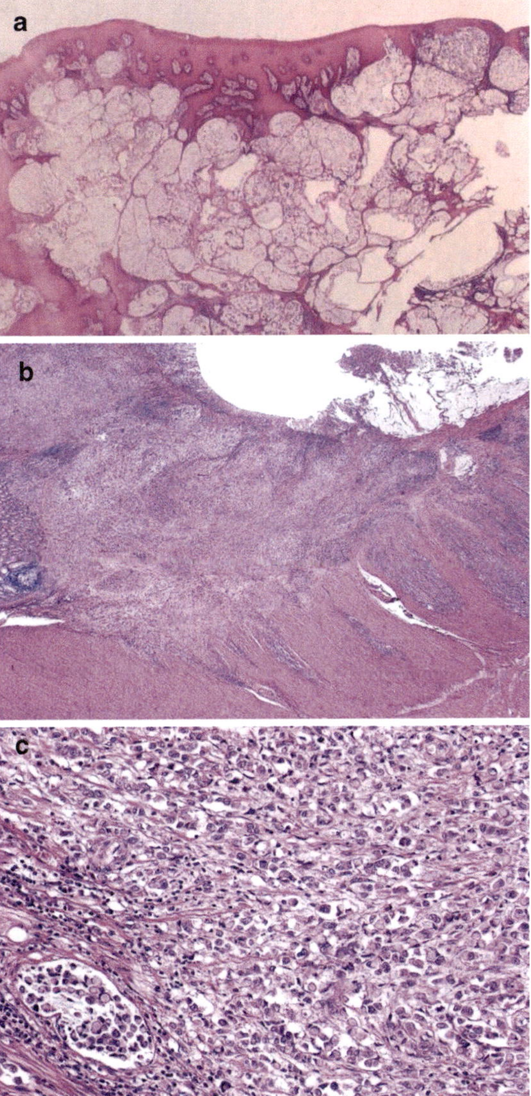

Fig. 27 H.E. staining: (**a**) Mucinous adenocarcinoma invading the skin adjacent to the anus. (**b**) Carcinoma invading the anorectal wall. (**c**) A poorly differentiated adenocarcinoma

6 Case 11: Carcinoma of the Lower Rectum and Anus Diagnosed by Anorectal Search Under Anesthesia due to Anal Pain and Mucus Stool

Kitaro Futami and Hiroshi Tanabe

40s, male, SL type, 12.5 years of illness

Onset in his 20s with perianal abscess, after which he was diagnosed with CD. Ten years after the onset, he underwent bowel resection and strictureplasty and was treated with biologics postoperatively. Three years after surgery, he had anal bleeding during defecation, increased frequency of stool, anal pain, and mucus stool. A close examination revealed a diagnosis of anorectal cancer, so magnetic resonance imaging, anorectal search, and colonoscopy were performed (Figs. 28, 29, and 30). A biopsy of the lesion showed poorly differentiated adenocarcinoma mixed with a mucinous component. Rectal wash cytology showed Class IV findings. CEA value: value: 0.2 ng/mL, CA19-9 value: 5.0 u/mL.

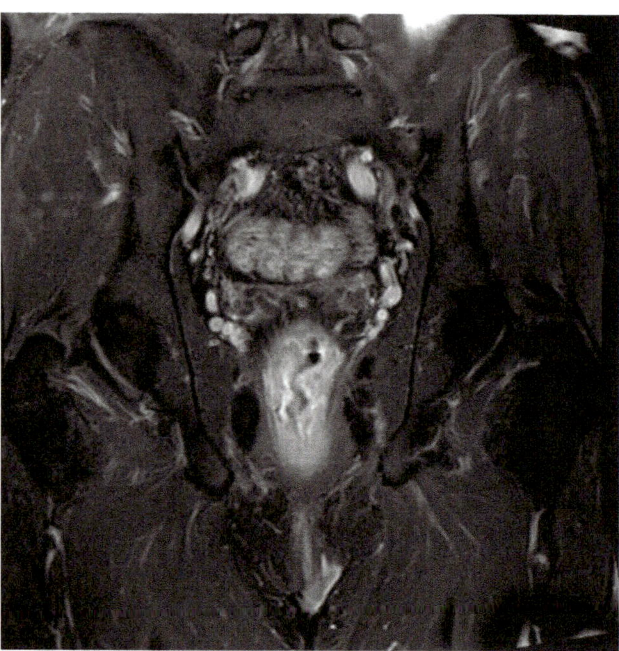

Fig. 28 MRI findings: Thickening of the wall of the lower rectum and anus

Surgery

Abdominoperineal resection, lymph node dissection, sigmoid colostomy

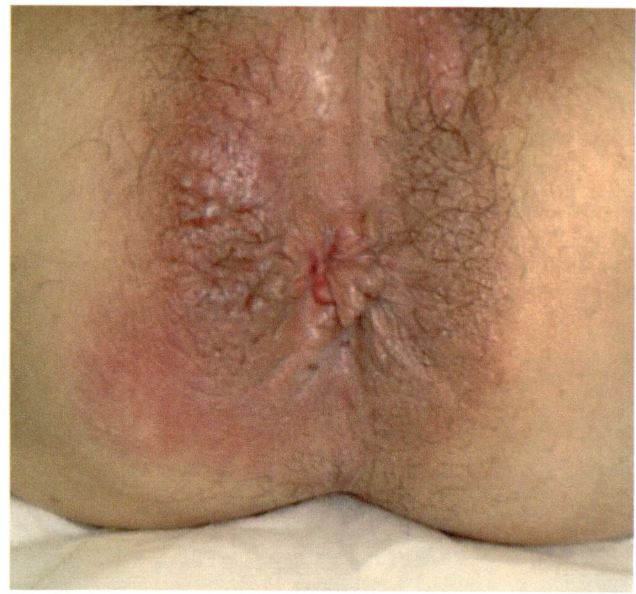

Fig. 29 Perianal findings: The perianal examination was performed under anesthesia because of the patient's serious perianal pain. There were no mass lesions on a visual examination, but painful perianal sclerosis and anal stenosis were remarked by palpation, and an anorectal mass lesion was found by a digital examination

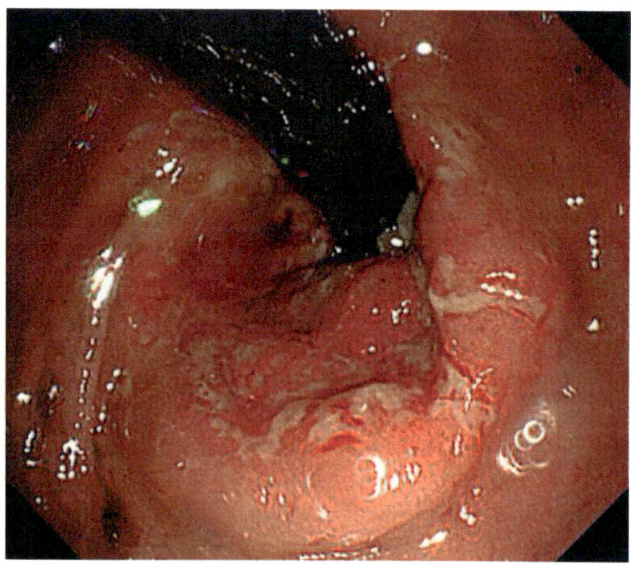

Fig. 30 Colonoscopy of retroflexion findings: Irregular ulcer lesion with a circumferential edge in the rectum and anus

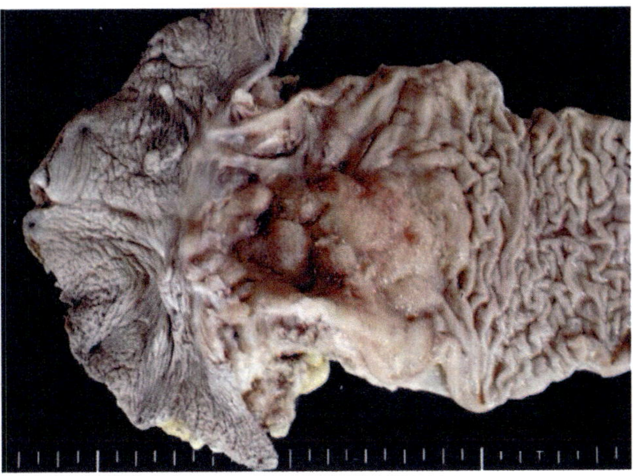

Fig. 31 Gross finding of the resected specimen: Irregular ulcerating invasive carcinoma was found occupying almost the lumen from the lower rectum and the anal canal

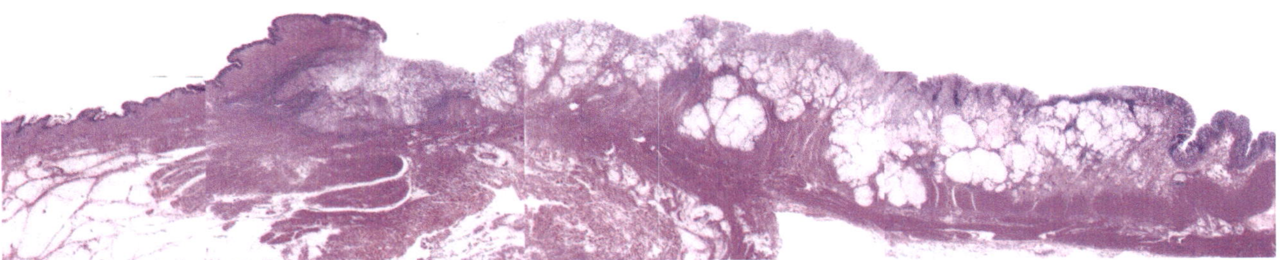

Fig. 32 Loupe finding: An advanced carcinoma invaded all layers of the anorectal wall

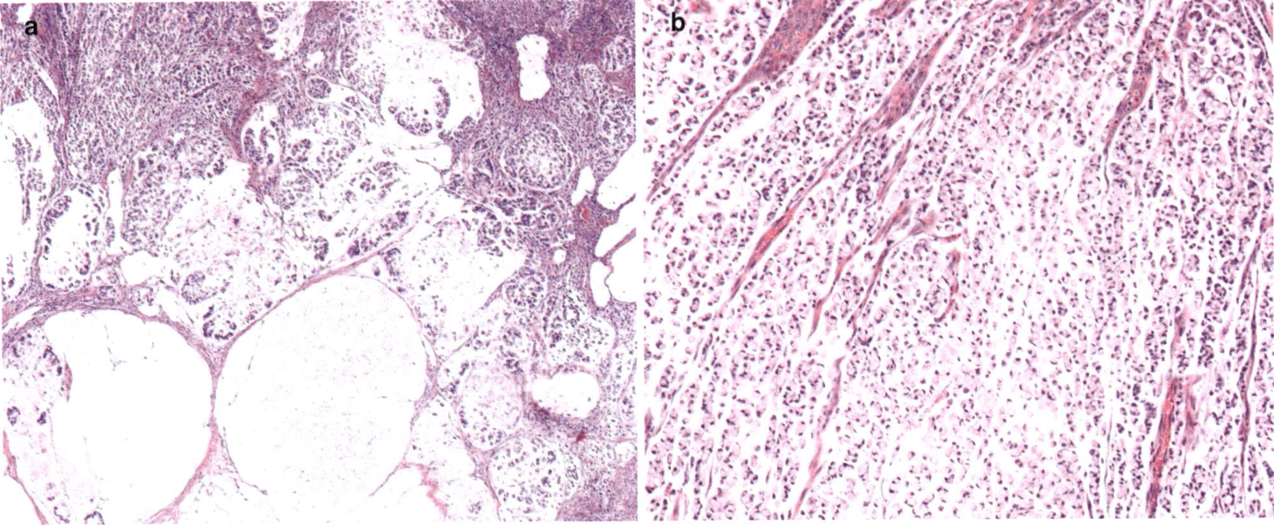

Fig. 33 H.E. staining: (**a**) The lesion was mainly poorly differentiated adenocarcinoma with intra- and extracellular mucous degeneration. (**b**) Close-up view of carcinoma

The Pathological Diagnosis

- Rectum and anal canal: Type 3, 70 mm, poorly differentiated adenocarcinoma with intra- and extracellular mucous degeneration (mucinous adenocarcinoma), pT4a (SE), Ly1c, V1a, INF c, Pn1a, pPM0, pDM0, pN1b.
- Stage IIIb: pT4a, pN1b, M0, P, H0, R0, Cur A.

Summary

Type 3 advanced mucinous adenocarcinoma was found occupying almost the entire lumen from the rectum (Rb) to the anal canal (Figs. 31, 32, and 33). Lymph node metastasis was also observed.

Mucinous adenocarcinoma of the rectum and anus is the most common cancer associated with Crohn's disease in Japan, and this case is a typical example.

7 Case 12: Lower Rectal and Anal Cancer Diagnosed by Retroflexion Endoscopy 20 Months After Detection of Atypical Epithelium in the Anal Canal

Kitaro Futami and Hiroshi Tanabe

30s, female, SL type, 17 years of illness

Onset in her teens, with an anal lesion diagnosed 4 years later. Five years after the diagnosis, she had repeated ileus. Because of ileal stricture and fistula to the ovary, she underwent the first ileal resection procedure. Four years after the surgery, recurrence was observed and a biologic agent was introduced. Four and a half years after her bowel surgery, she underwent an anal procedure (anal dilation and seton drainage with a biopsy) under anesthesia for cancer surveillance, and atypical epithelium was detected. After that, endoscopic observation was performed every few months, and 1 year and 8 months after the detection of the atypical epithelium, an endoscopic examination revealed a villous tumor in the anal canal (Fig. 34a–d). A biopsy revealed a very well-differentiated adenocarcinoma. No obvious cancer findings were detected on CT examination (Fig. 35). In addition, FDG-PET showed no accumulation in the cancer lesion. During this period, her anorectal symptoms did not change. CEA value: value: 0.6 ng/mL, CA19-9 value: 6.0 u/mL.

Surgery

Abdominoperineal resection, lymph node dissection, transverse colostomy

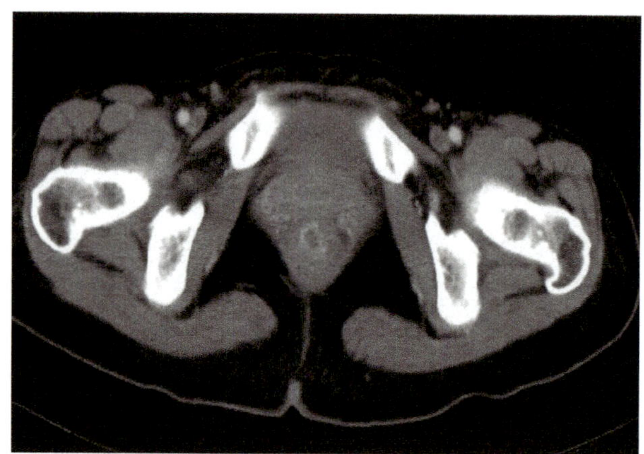

Fig. 35 CT findings: No evidence of tumor in the anal canal, no distant metastasis, no enlarged lymph nodes

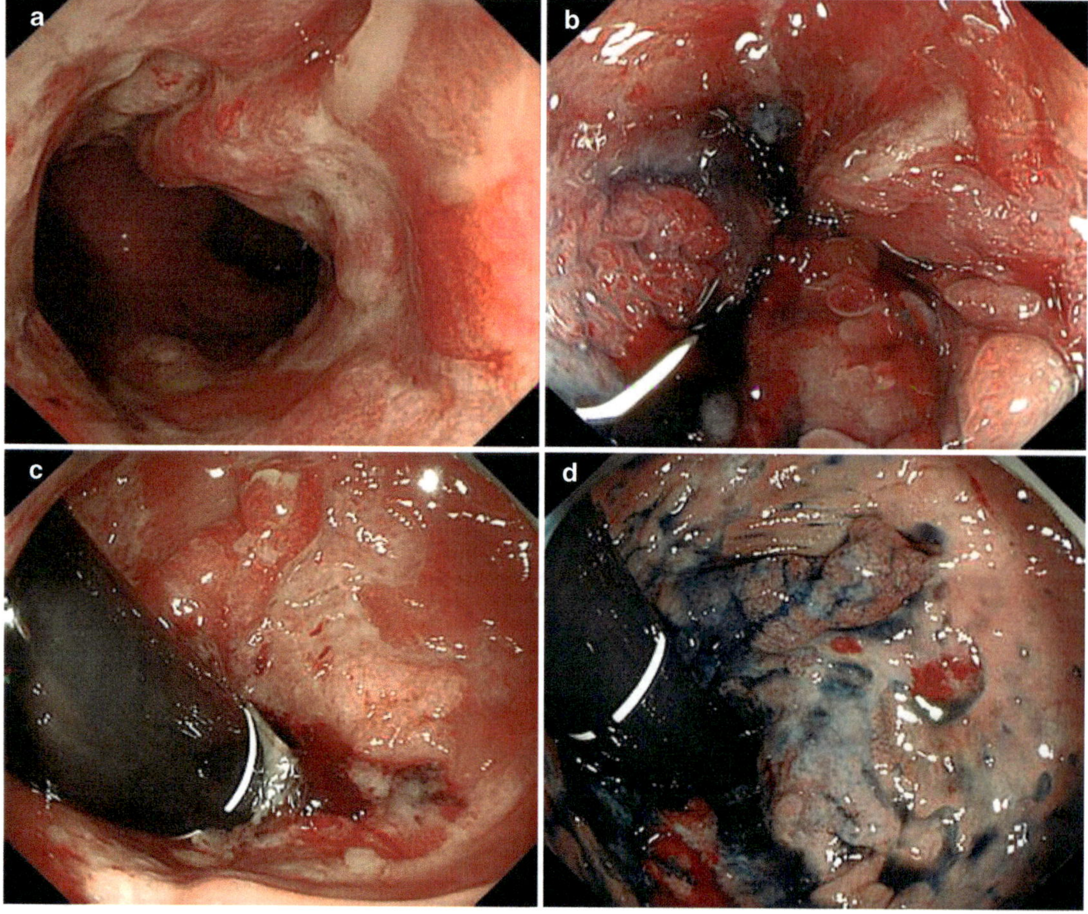

Fig. 34 Colonoscopy findings: (**a** and **b**) Forward view: Erythematous villous tumor in the anal canal. (**c** and **d**) Retroflexion view: With and without dye-spreading showed the cancer lesion much clear

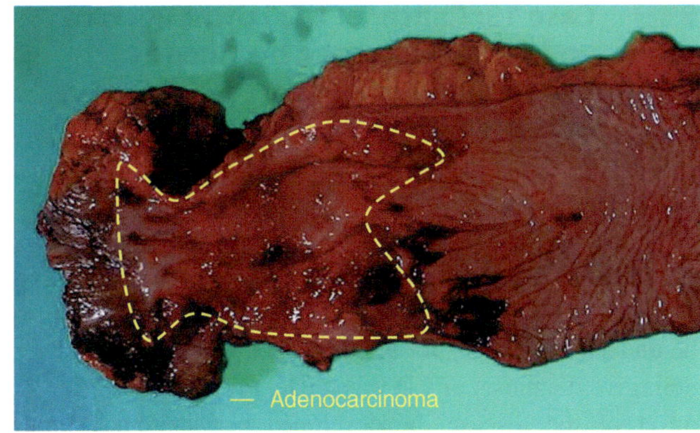

Fig. 36 Gross finding of the resected specimen: A type 5 advanced carcinoma was found occupying the entire lumen from the rectum (Rb) to the anal canal and delineation of invasion by yellow line

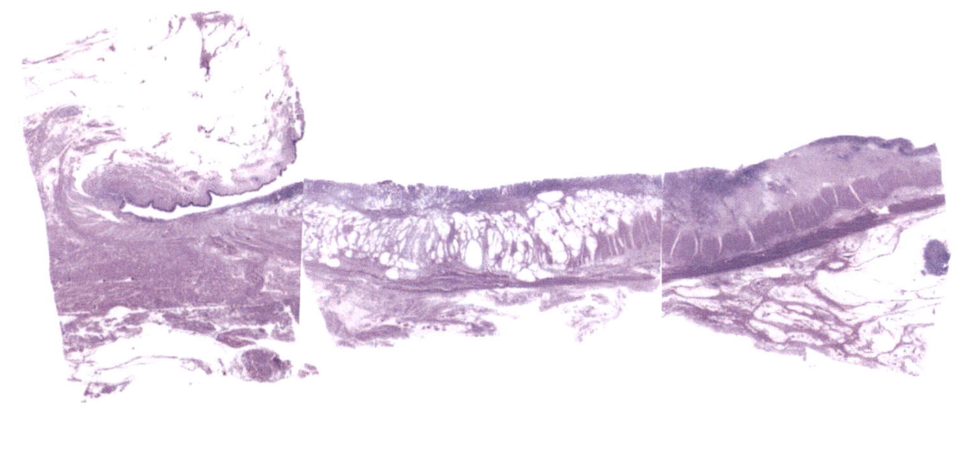

Fig. 37 Loupe finding. The depth of the lesion was invasive to the adventitia of the rectum

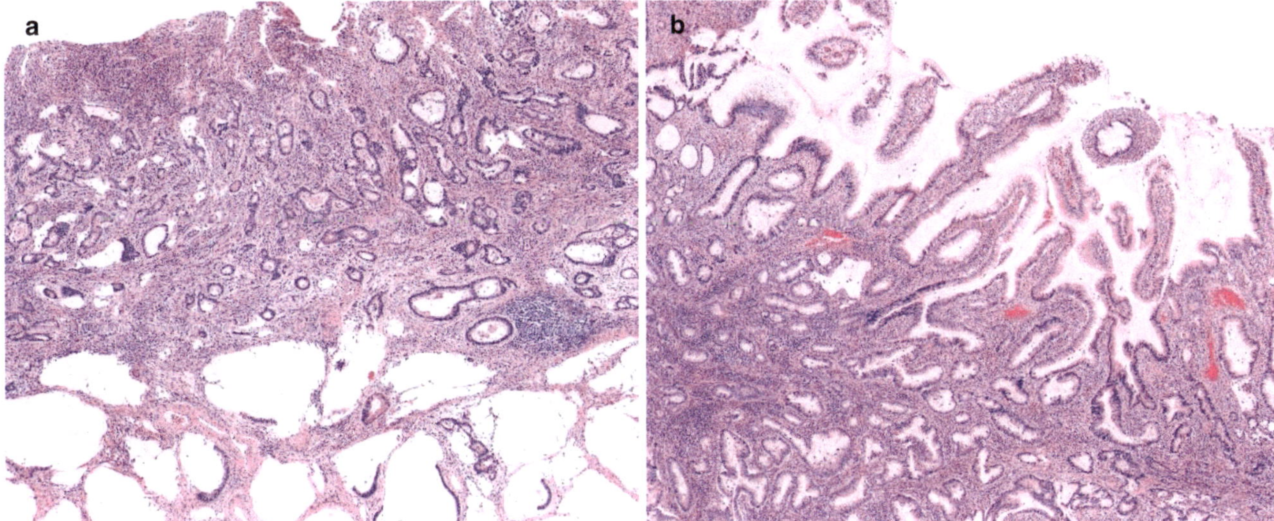

Fig. 38 H.E. staining: (**a**) The tumor was a mucinous adenocarcinoma composed mainly of well-differentiated tubular adenocarcinoma. (**b**) In a part very well-differentiated adenocarcinoma was found in some superficial layers

The Pathological Diagnosis

- Rectum and anal canal: Type 5, 50 mm, very well- to well-differentiated adenocarcinoma with extracellular mucous degeneration (mucinous adenocarcinoma), pT3 (A), Ly1a, V1a, BD1, INF b, Pn1a, pPM0, pDM0, pRM0, pN0.
- Stage IIa, pT3, pN0, M0, P0, H0, R0, Cur A.

Summary

Type 5 advanced mucinous adenocarcinoma was found occupying almost the entire lumen from the rectum (Rb) to the anal canal (Figs. 36, 37, and 38) without lymph node metastasis. Retroflexion-view endoscopy was effective for diagnosing anal canal cancer in this case.

8 Case 13: Cancer of the Lower Rectum and Anus Diagnosed by Mucus Discharge After 15 Years of Exclusion of the Rectum

Kitaro Futami and Hiroshi Tanabe

50s, male, SL type, 30 years of illness

Onset in his 20s with abdominal symptom. One year later, he underwent surgery for perianal fistula. Four years later, a definitive diagnosis of CD was made. Fifteen years after the onset of the disease, he developed perianal and scrotal abscesses and anorectal stenosis and was referred to our hospital. He underwent bowel resection and sigmoid colostomy with exclusion of the rectum, after which the colostomy was not closed, and he was observed with conventional medication. Fifteen years after the colostomy, he visited the surgeon complaining of mucus discharge from his anus (Fig. 39). Mucinous adenocarcinoma was diagnosed by a transanal search under anesthesia and simultaneous colonoscopy (Fig. 40). No cancer findings were detected on MRI (Fig. 41). CEA value: 1.9 ng/mL, CA19-9 value: 5.5 u/mL.

Surgery

1. Abdominoperineal resection, lymph node dissection, combined resection of the left seminal vesicle, and descending colostomy
2. Right hemicolectomy, end-to-end anastomosis, and jejunal stricture formation for CD.

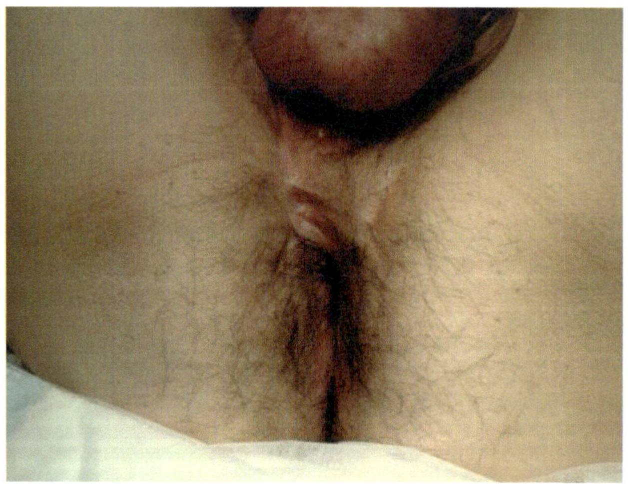

Fig. 39 Perianal findings: Sclerotic, tender, and stenotic perianal region; a digital examination was not possible in an outpatient setting

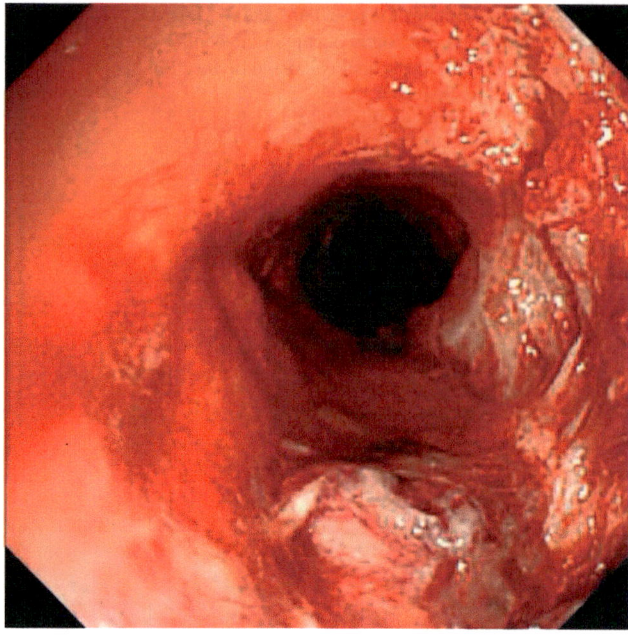

Fig. 40 Colonoscopy findings: Irregular elevated lesion in the rectum and anus

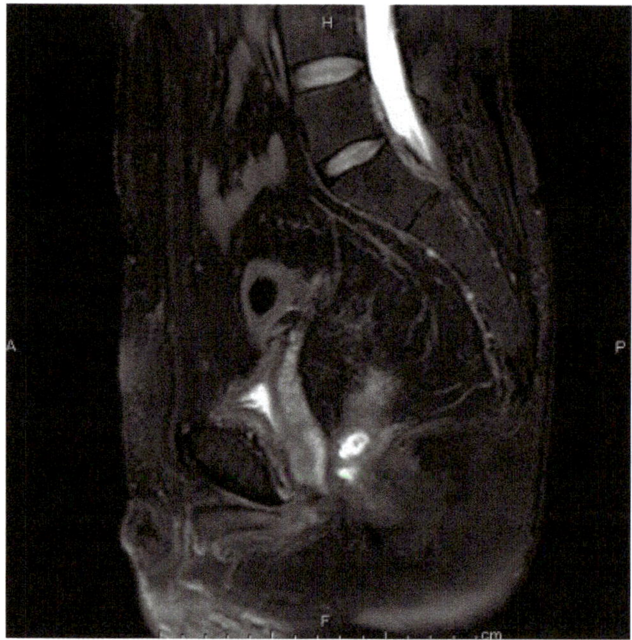

Fig. 41 MRI findings: No cancerous lesions detected

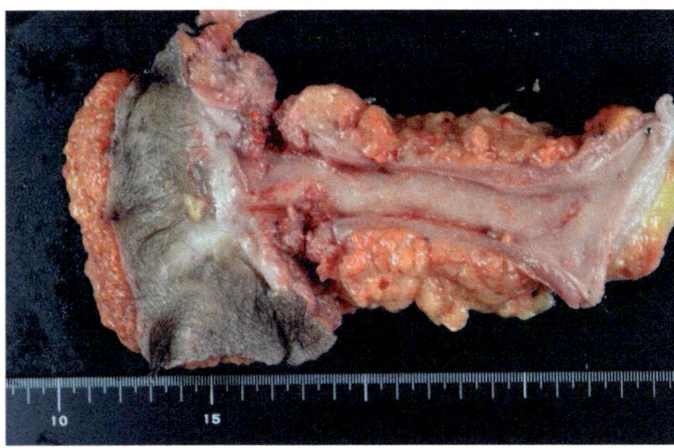

Fig. 42 Gross findings of resected specimen: Type 5 cancer was found on the site of lower rectum (Rb) and anus

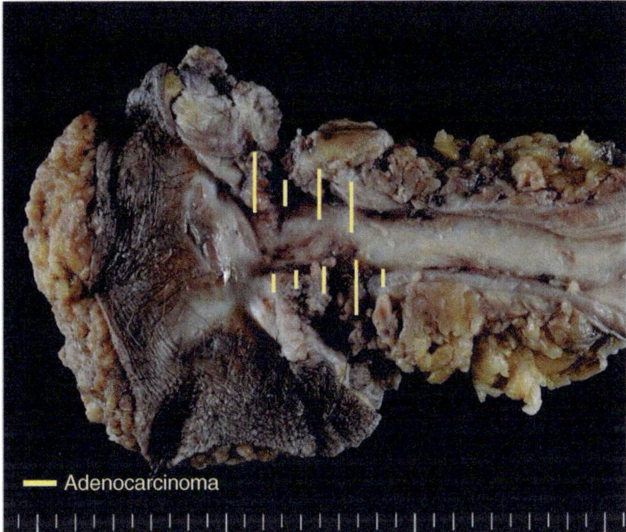

Fig. 43 Close-up view and demonstration of cancer invasion: The cancer lesion was presented in yellow line and occupied about half of the lumen

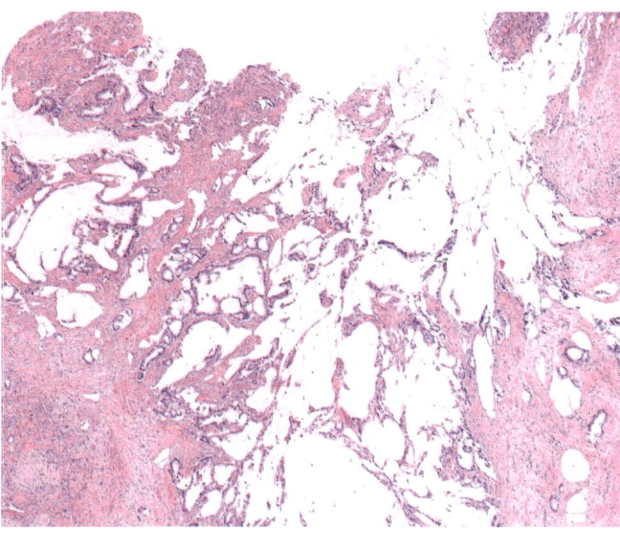

Fig. 44 H.E. staining: The lesion was a well-differentiated tubular adenocarcinoma with partly extracellular mucous degeneration and have invaded the adventitia of the rectum

The Pathological Diagnosis

- Rectum and anal canal: Type 5, 35 mm, very well- to well-differentiated adenocarcinoma with partly extracellular mucinous degeneration, pT3 (A), Ly0, V1a, BD1, INF b, Pn1b, pPM0, pDM0, pRM0, pN0.
- Stage IIa: pT3, pN0, M0, P0, H0, R0, Cur A.

Summary

Type 5 advanced cancer was presented on the site of lower rectum (Rb) and anus and occupied about half of the lumen (Figs. 42, 43, and 44). The carcinoma has invaded the adventitia of the rectum, but there were no lymph node metastases. A periodic examination of the excluded rectum and anus is mandatory, even if there are no symptoms due to stoma.

9 Case 14: Cancer of the Lower Rectum and Anus Diagnosed During Endoscopy for Ileocolonic Anastomotic Dilation Therapy

Kitaro Futami and Hiroshi Tanabe

50s, male, SL type, 30 years of illness

Onset in his 20s with ileus. He was diagnosed 1 year later and started medical therapy. Four years after the onset of the disease, he underwent anal surgery and the first bowel resection procedure. Thereafter, he was treated with medication as appropriate. In the course of his treatment, he underwent bowel surgery three times in total, had multiple flare-ups of perirectal fistula, and developed anal stenosis, so dilation therapy was performed as needed. Twenty-four years and six months after the first surgery, he underwent an anal procedure under anesthesia, and a biopsy of the mucosa of the anal canal revealed inflammatory findings. On follow-up CT examination, no cancerous findings were detected (Fig. 45a, b). Six months later, during an endoscopic examination for dilation of ileocolonic anastomotic stricture, a villous tumor of the lower rectum was found (Fig. 46a, b), and a biopsy revealed a diagnosis of well-differentiated adenocarcinoma. There were no anorectal symptoms during this period. CEA value: 1.7 ng/mL, CA19-9 value: 2.0 u/mL.

Surgery

1. Abdominoperineal resection, lymph node dissection, ileostomy
2. Ileocolonic exclusion bypass for CD

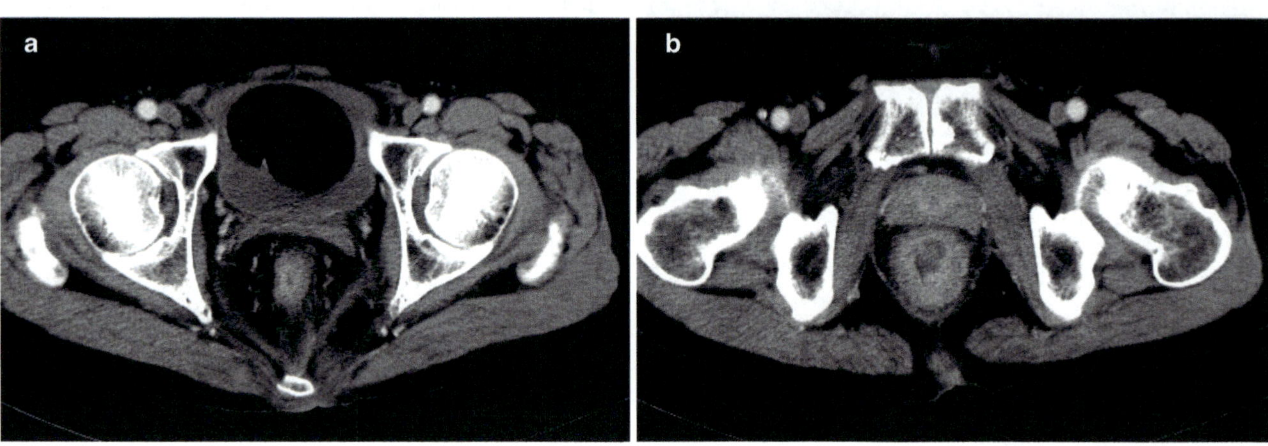

Fig. 45 CT findings: (**a**) Diffuse inflammation was observed in the upper rectum. (**b**) The cancerous site of the lower rectum was visualized as inflammation

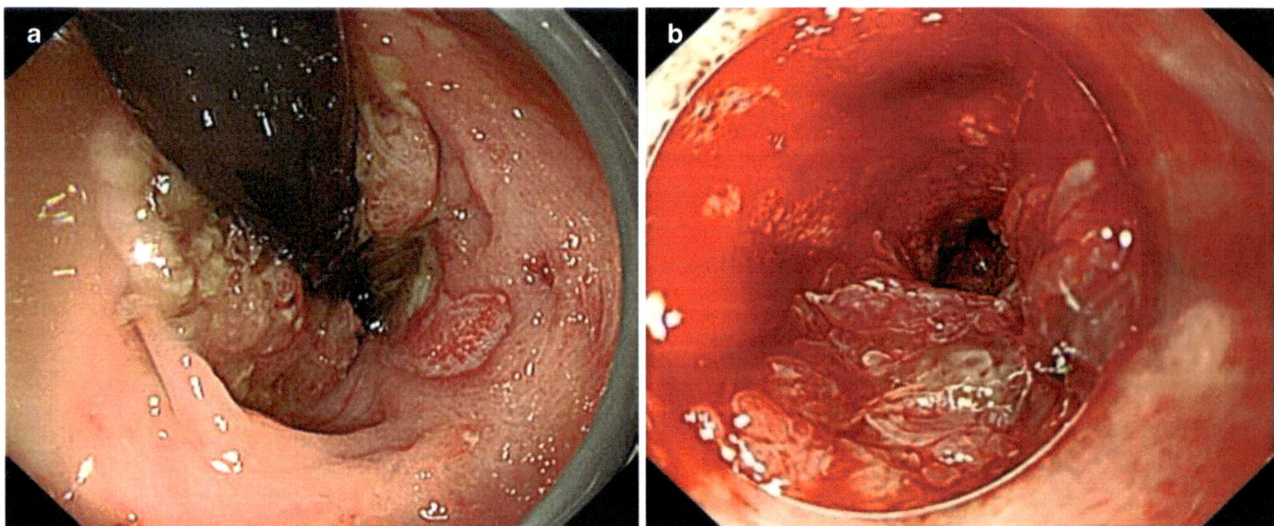

Fig. 46 Colonoscopy images: (**a**) Retroflexion endoscopy showed a circumferential villous tumor, and the boundary of the lesion was detected in the lower rectum. (**b**) Circumscribed villous tumor of the lower rectum to the anus

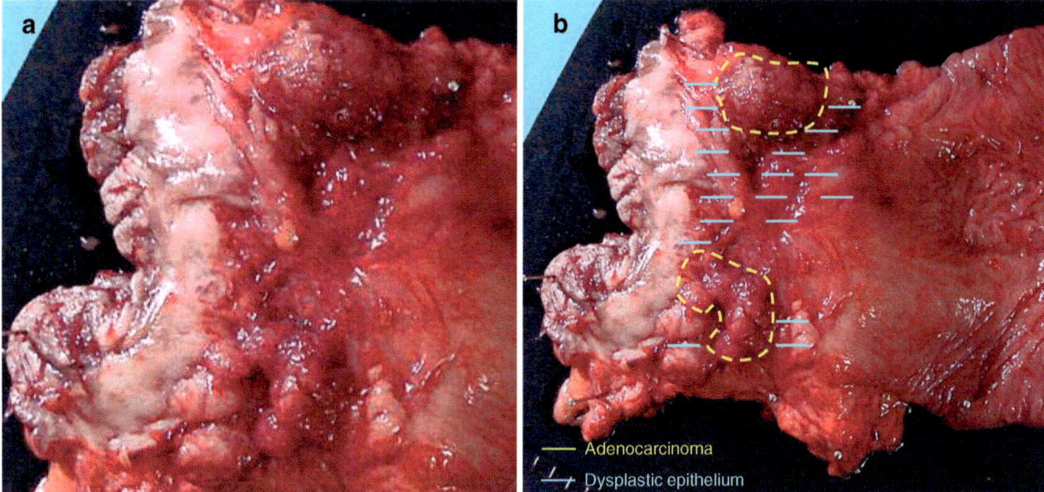

Fig. 47 Gross finding and schematic illustration of various tumor extensions of the resected specimen: (**a**) A raised lesion with a partially villous surface was found from the rectum (Rb) to the anal canal. (**b**) Adenocarcinoma was shown in yellow line and dysplastic epithelium was shown in blue line

Fig. 48 Loupe finding. A raised lesion with a partially villous surface was found from the rectum (Rb) to the anal canal. The carcinoma have invaded the adventitia of the rectum. This lesion was located near the fistula (arrow), but there was no tumor invasion into the fistula

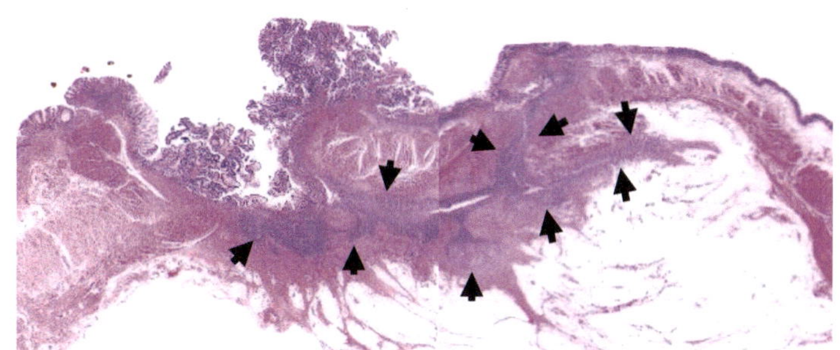

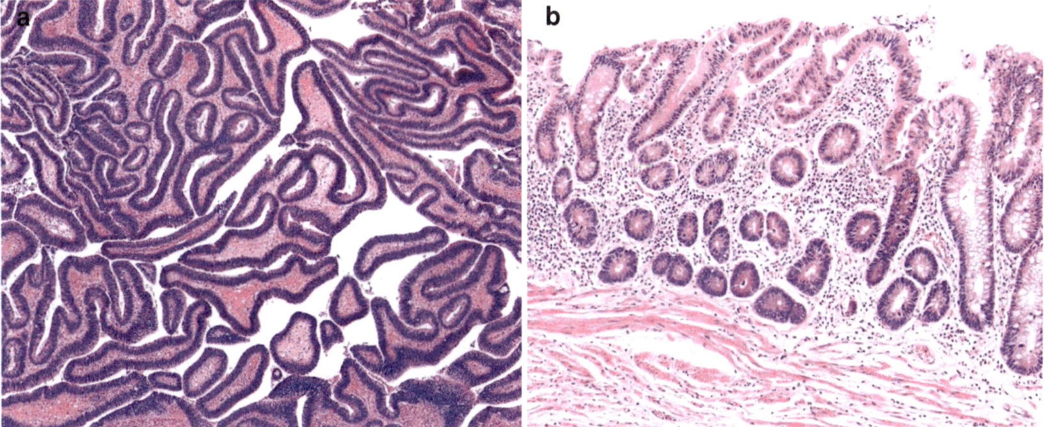

Fig. 49 H.E. staining: (**a**) Tubulovillous well-differentiated adenocarcinoma was found. (**b**) A dysplastic epithelium was found in the surrounding area

The Pathological Diagnosis

- Rectum and anal canal: Type I-like advanced, 35 mm, very well- to well-differentiated adenocarcinoma (Figs. 47, 48, and 49) with dysplastic epithelium (Fig. 49b), pT3 (A), Ly0, V0, BD1, INF a, Pn0, pPM0, pDM0, pRM0, pN0.
- Stage IIa: pT3, pN0, M0, P0, H0, R0, Cur A.

Summary

Type I-like advanced cancer was found from the rectum (Rb) to the anal canal (Fig. 47). The carcinoma has invaded the adventitia of the rectum. This lesion was located near the fistula (arrow), but there was no tumor invasion into the fistula (Figs. 48 and 49).

The tumor was not recognized by a digital rectal examination, but endoscopy, especially the retroflexion view, was effective in this case.

10 Case 15: Cancer of the Anal Canal Diagnosed by Endoscopic Biopsies from a Skin Tag and a Refractory Wound After Resection

Kitaro Futami and Hiroshi Tanabe

50s, female, SL type, 42 years of illness

Onset in her teens with abdominal symptoms. Nine years later, she was diagnosed with CD. During therapies, she underwent three intestinal resection procedures, followed by resection of an anal skin tag. Twenty-eight years after the first surgery, bleeding on defecation was noted. Perianal lesions were noted: an enlarged skin tag at the 12 o'clock position and a vulvar fistula at the 1 o'clock position, along with anal stenosis (Fig. 50). Under anesthesia, resection of the skin tag and a biopsy of the anal polyp were performed, but no atypia was detected. Four months later, she complained of anal pain, and an outpatient biopsy revealed atypical epithelium with positive p53 staining at the previous excision site (Fig. 51). A reexamination by colonoscopy (Fig. 52) and biopsy detected mucinous adenocarcinoma. Preoperative MRI showed an unclear mass lesion on the wall of the anal canal (Fig. 53).

Surgery

1. Abdominoperineal resection, lymph node dissection combined resection of posterior wall of the vagina, descending colostomy
2. ileocolonic resection, end-to-end anastomosis for CD lesions

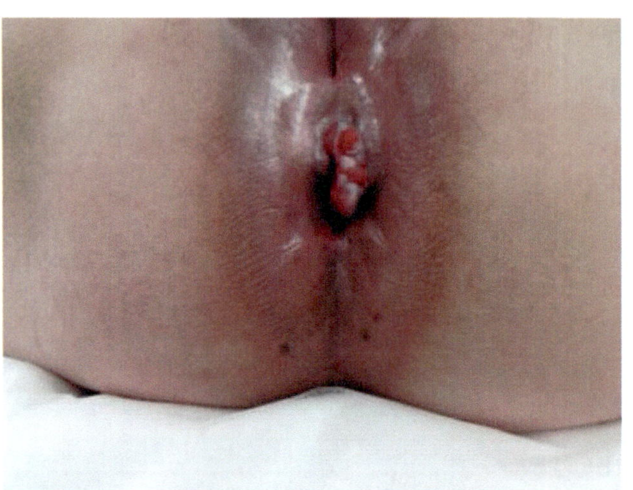

Fig. 50 Perianal findings: Tense skin tag on the anterior wall

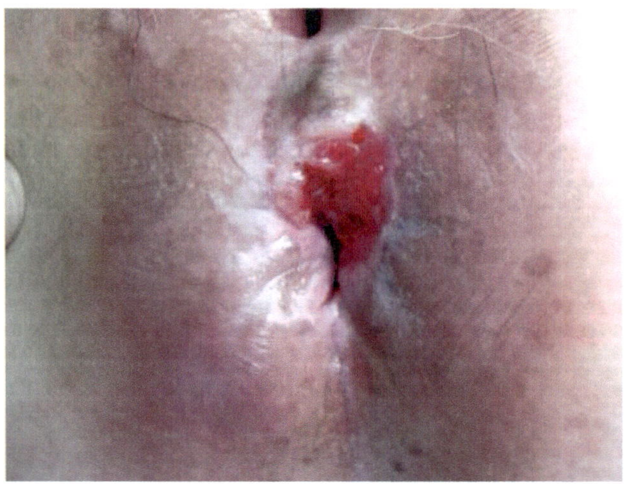

Fig. 51 Perianal findings after skin tag resection: Healed reddish granulation at the site of skin tag excision. (This figure is quoted from the literature below; Figure 2 in Futami K, et al. Current Surgical Strategy for Perianal Crohn's Disease. J. Jpn Soc. Coloproctol. 2017; 70: 624)

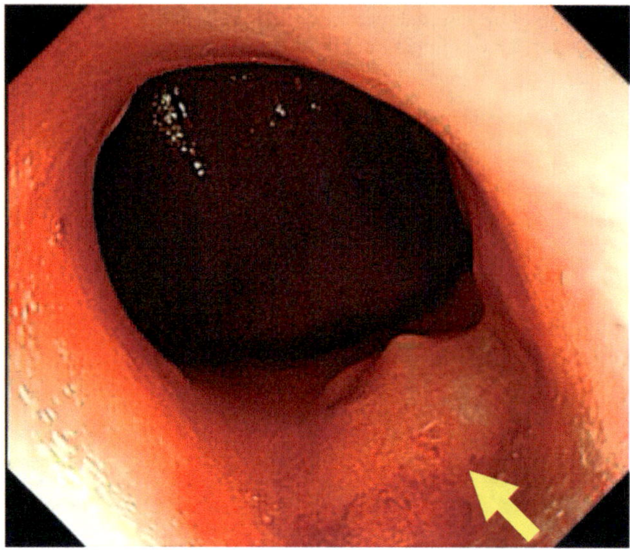

Fig. 52 Colonoscopy findings: A firm mass at the right anterior wall and a depressed lesion in the anal canal

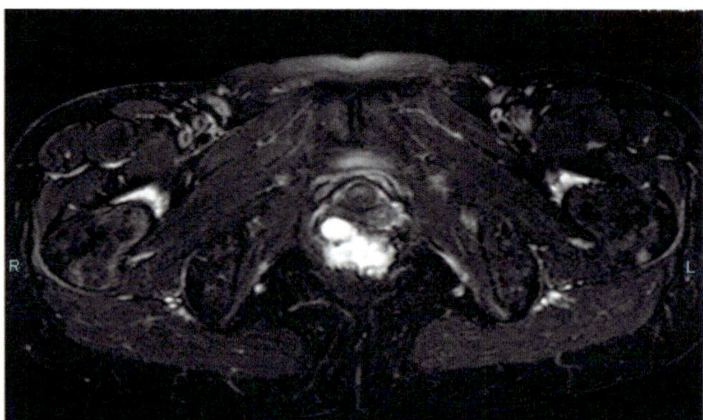

Fig. 53 MRI findings: Mass on the right anterior wall of the anal canal showing an unclear boundary with the vagina

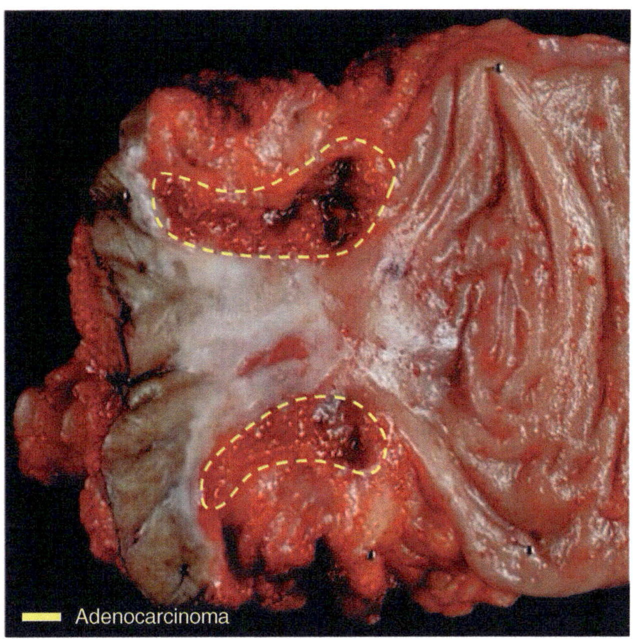

Fig. 54 Gross finding of the resected specimen: A semicircular type 5 advanced carcinoma with the locus of the lesion in the anal canal was noted (yellow line)

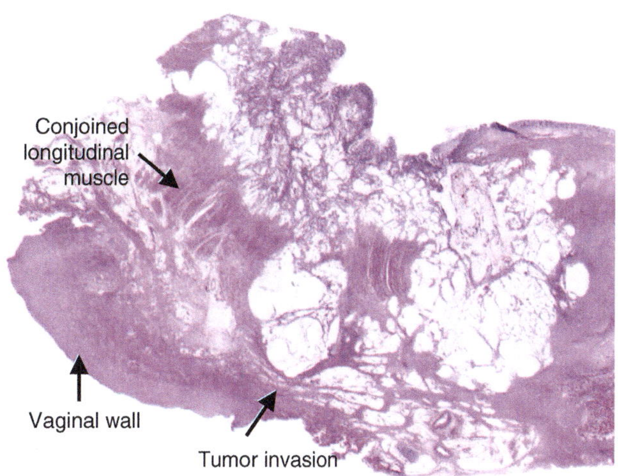

Fig. 55 Loupe finding: The mucinous adenocarcinoma has invaded the rectovaginal septum beyond the conjoined longitudinal muscle

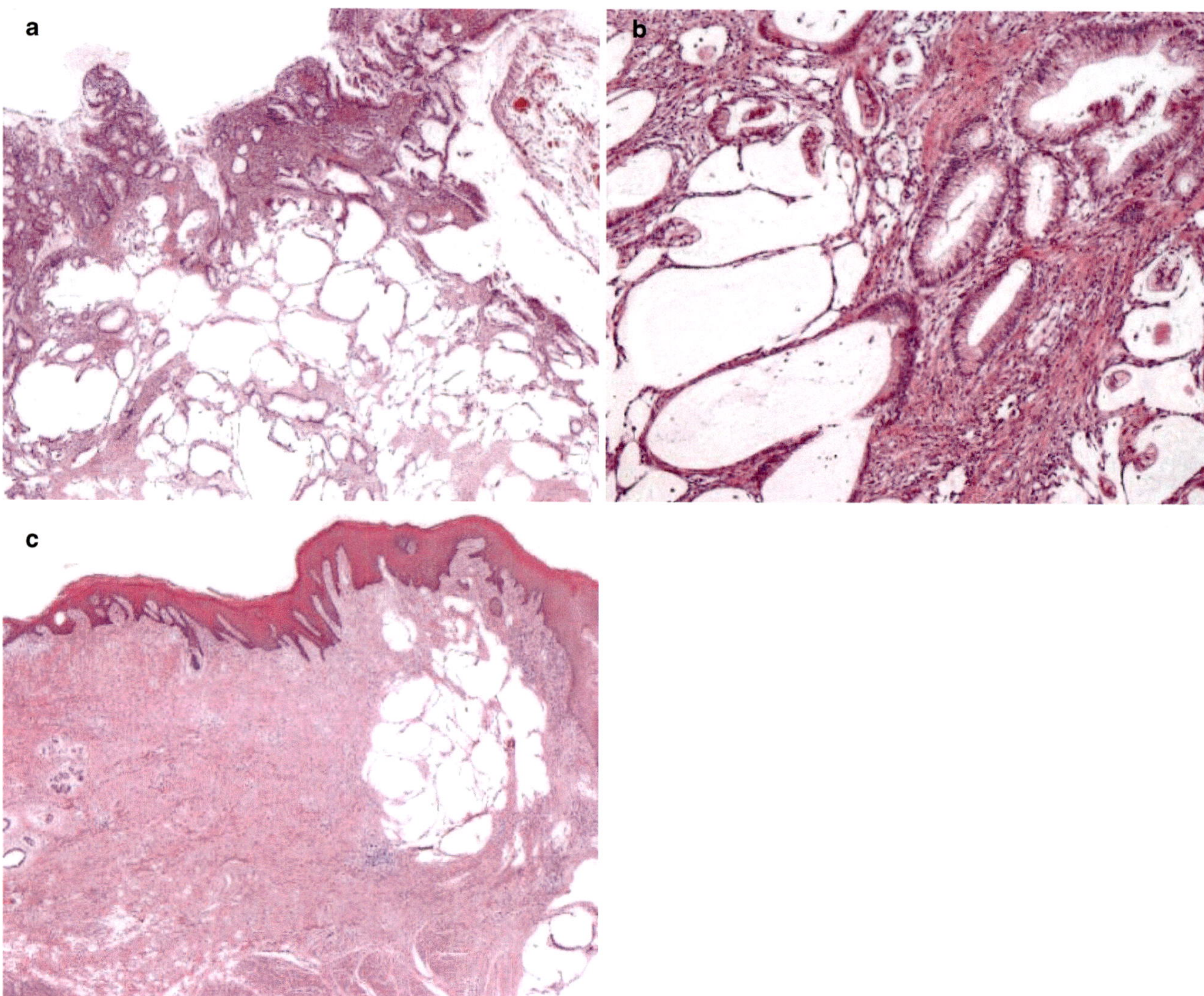

Fig. 56 H.E. staining of the carcinoma: (**a** and **b**) The lesion was mucinous adenocarcinoma consisting of very well- to poorly differentiated adenocarcinoma of the rectal type. (**c**) On the anorectal side, tumor cells were found to have invaded the perianal skin

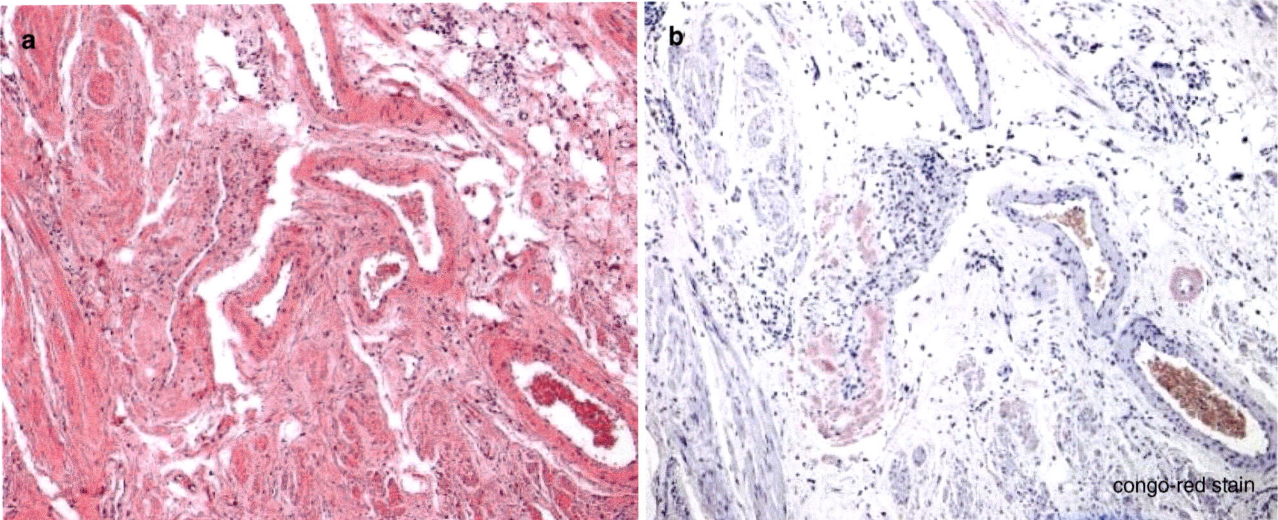

Fig. 57 The findings of amyloid deposition: (**a**) H.E. staining, there was a mild deposition of AA amyloid in the surrounding vessel wall. (**b**) Congo-red stain showing AA amyloidosis and the patient had secondary amyloidosis

The Pathological Diagnosis

- Anal canal: Type 5, 45 mm, very well- to poorly differentiated adenocarcinoma of rectal type with extracellular mucous degeneration (mucinous adenocarcinoma), pT3, Ly1a, V1a, Pn1a, pPM0, pDM0, pRM0, pN0, associated with secondary amyloidosis.
- Stage IIa: pT3, pN0, M0, P0, H0, R0, Cur A.

Summary

Type 5 advanced mucinous adenocarcinoma has located in the anal canal (Figs. 54, 55, and 56). In addition, the finding of secondary amyloidosis was found (Fig. 57). The patient was suspected of having cancer due to postoperative wound failure in the anus.

11 Case 16: Anal Canal Cancer Diagnosed by Biopsy from Aggressive Anal Ulcer 7 Years After Diagnosis of Anal Fissure

Kitaro Futami and Hiroshi Tanabe

40s, female, SL type, 23.4 years of illness

Onset in her 20s with abdominal pain and diarrhea. She was diagnosed soon after, and medical therapy was started. Seven years later, she underwent bowel surgery, and a skin tag was diagnosed 8 years after surgery, so medical therapy was added at the time of recurrence. Perianal fistula and anal fissure were diagnosed the following year. Fifteen years after the initial bowel surgery, reoperation with bowel resection was performed. Postoperatively, she was observed with medical therapy, and the CEA level remained high (5.0–10.0 ng/mL). Ten months after the second surgery, bleeding on defecation from an enlarged ulcer lesion at the 6 o'clock position was noted, and tenderness was exacerbated. One year and 2 months after the second surgery, the ulcer lesion at the 6 o'clock position in the anus had grown further, and sclerosis of the lesion was observed on palpation (Fig. 58). Because of increased pain, a biopsy was performed in the outpatient setting under local anesthesia, and a diagnosis of well-differentiated adenocarcinoma and Class IIIb rectal wash cytology was made. No evidence of cancer was detected on preoperative imaging examinations (Fig. 59). CEA value: 10.8 ng/mL, CA19-9 value: 23.0 u/mL.

Surgery

Abdominoperineal resection, lymph node dissection, sigmoid colostomy.

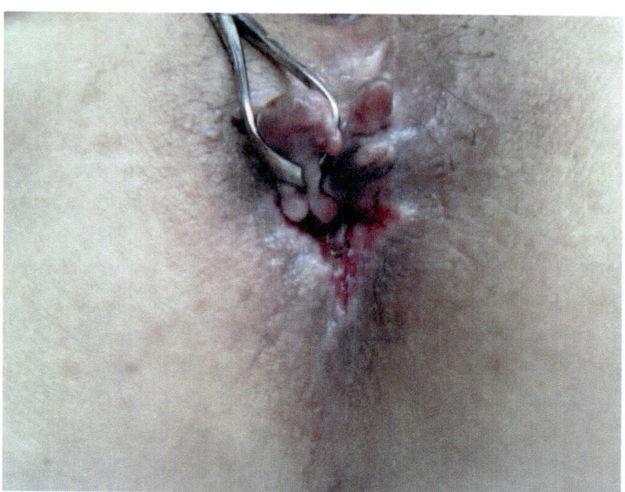

Fig. 58 Perianal findings: Enlarged ulcer lesion at the 6 o'clock position (observed by grasping the skin tag). She was diagnosed by an outpatient biopsy

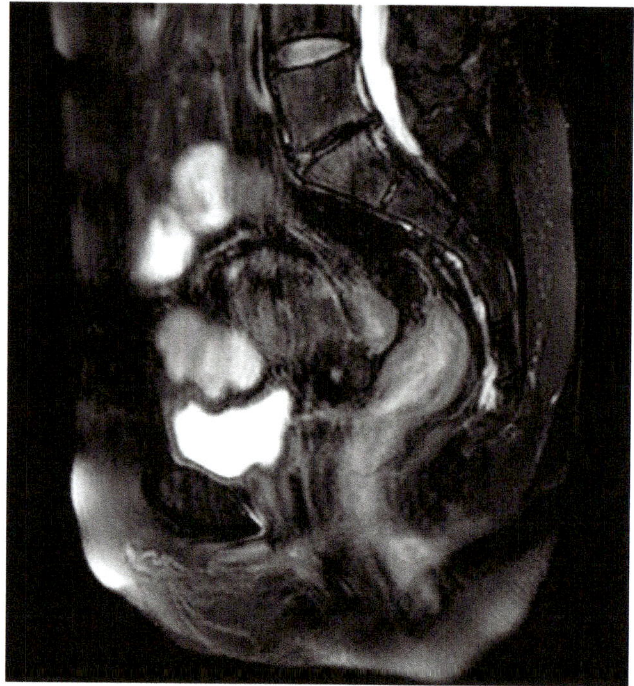

Fig. 59 MRI findings: Edematous changes in the soft tissues of the anal canal with no evidence of cancer. No other imaging findings depicted cancerous lesions

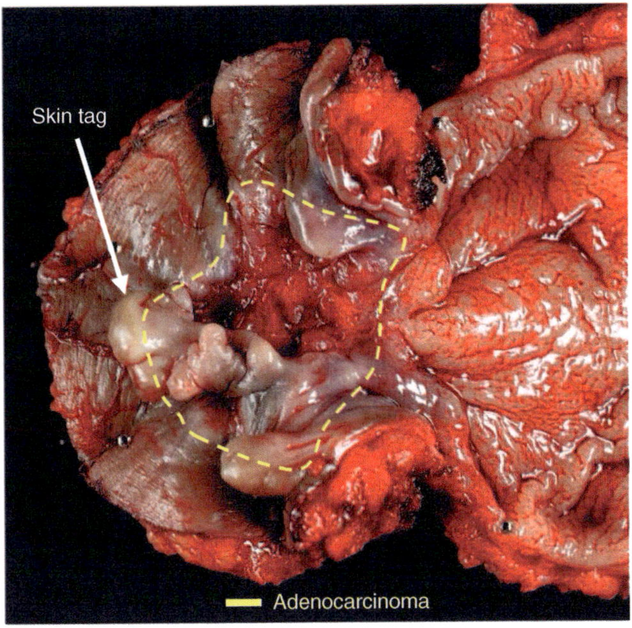

Fig. 60 Gross finding of the resected specimen: Skin tag and cancer extension were shown in yellow line. The lesion was located at the anal canal and occupied approximately 2/3 of the circumference of the canal, forming type 2 advanced cancer

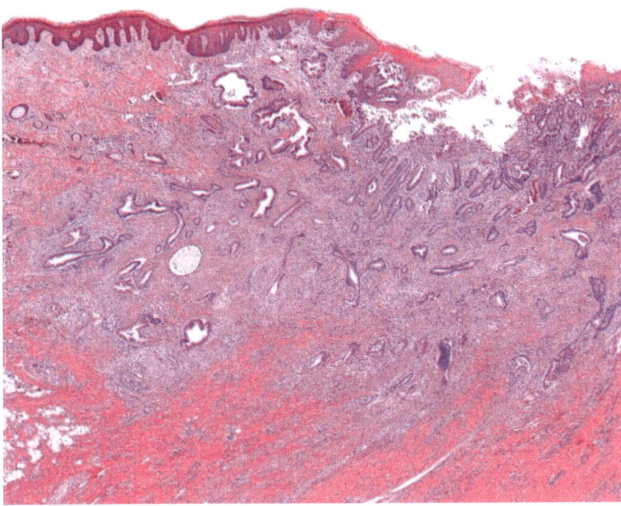

Fig. 62 H.E. staining: The lesion was a rectal-type well-differentiated tubular adenocarcinoma. On the anorectal side, there was invasion into the dermis of the perianal skin

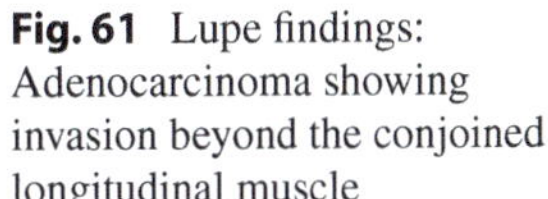

Fig. 61 Lupe findings: Adenocarcinoma showing invasion beyond the conjoined longitudinal muscle

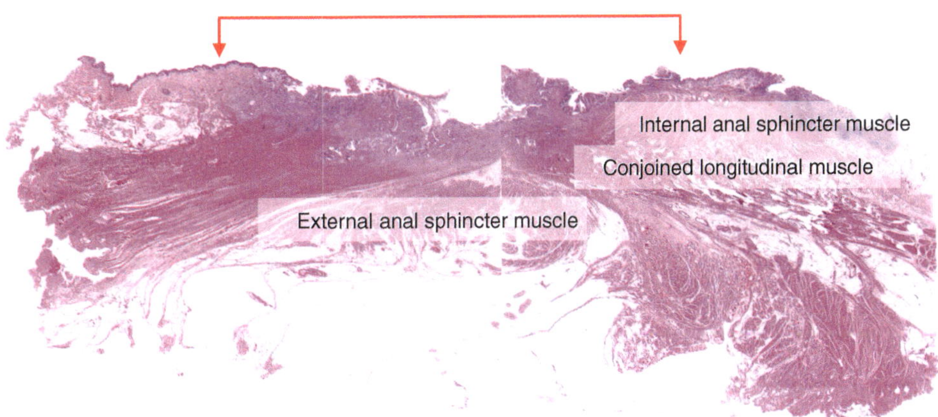

The Pathological Diagnosis

- Anal canal: Type 2, well- to moderately differentiated adenocarcinoma of rectal type, pT3, Ly0, V0, BD1, Pn0, pPM0, pDM0, pRM0, pN0.
- Stage IIa: pT3, pN0, M0, P0, H0, R0, Cur A.

Summary

Type 2 advanced adenocarcinoma of rectal type in the anal canal (Figs. 60, 61, and 62) without lymph node metastasis. When an anal ulcer lesion worsens during the disease course, cancer should be suspected.

12 Case 17: Anal Cancer Diagnosed by Surveillance Biopsy of Perianal Fistula

Kitaro Futami and Hiroshi Tanabe

60s, female, SL type, 16.2 years of illness

Onset in her 40s with abdominal symptoms. CD was diagnosed and medical therapy was started. Eight years later, exacerbation of abdominal symptoms (stenosis, internal fistula) and perianal abscess were noted. She was thus referred to our hospital for surgery and underwent her first bowel surgery. Perianal abscess incision and drainage by the seton method were performed, followed by continued medical treatment. She underwent intestinal surgeries three times, along with multiple seton drainage procedures and biopsies of the anal region (no atypical epithelium detected). Biologics were introduced after the third intestinal surgery, and 1 year and 6 months later, perianal abscess and fistula flared up (Fig. 63), so seton drainage was performed again. Biopsies of the fistula at the 5 o'clock position showed mucinous adenocarcinoma (Fig. 64). The abdominoperineal resection including perianal fistulas was performed (Fig. 65).

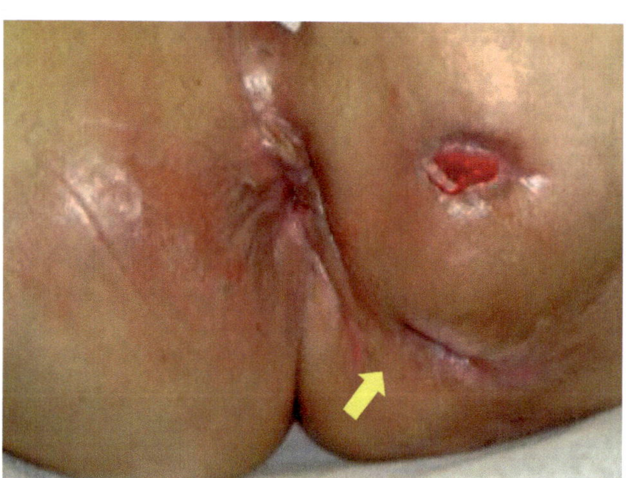

Fig. 63 Perianal findings: Left side of the perianal area, semicircular multiple fistulas. Biopsy site was shown in arrow

Surgery

Abdominoperineal resection, lymph node dissection, sigmoid colostomy.

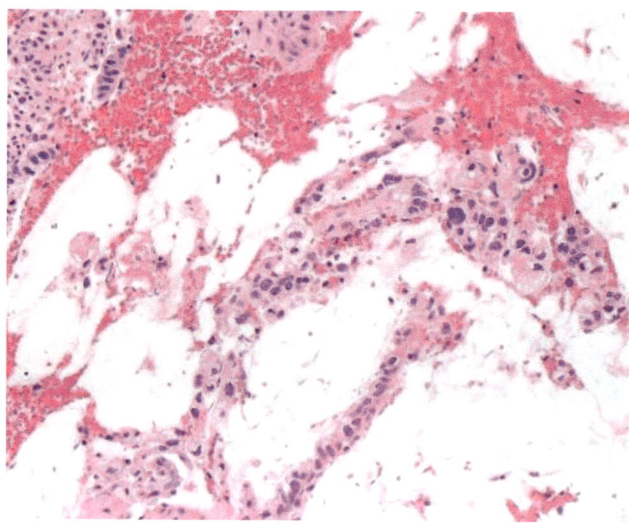

Fig. 64 Histological findings of biopsy: Mucinous adenocarcinoma was found in the biopsy from perianal fistula

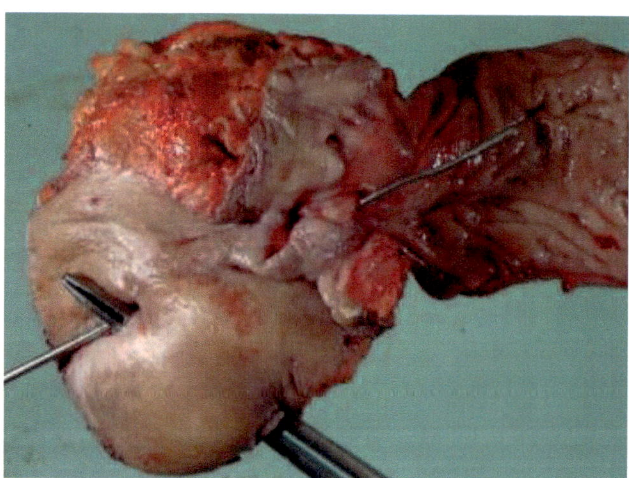

Fig. 65 Resected specimen: A long fistulous tract penetrating by a wire

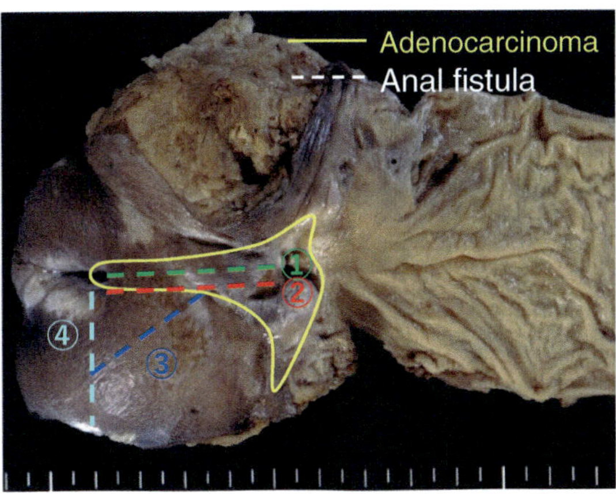

Fig. 66 Macroscopic finding and schematic illustration of extension of cancer in connection with fistulous tract: Adenocarcinoma was shown in yellow line and four fistulous tracts (①, ②, ③, ④) were shown in dotted four lines

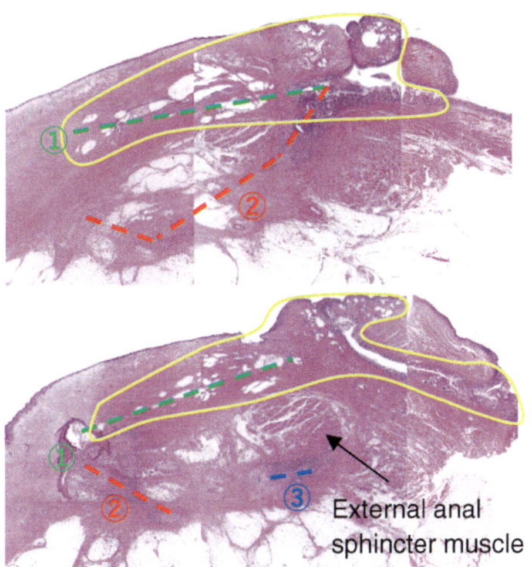

Fig. 67 Lupe findings: Two complicated fistulae were formed from the anal canal to the perianal skin (①, ②). Adenocarcinoma has grown along the course of the fistula ① (yellow line), suggesting that it originated from the fistula

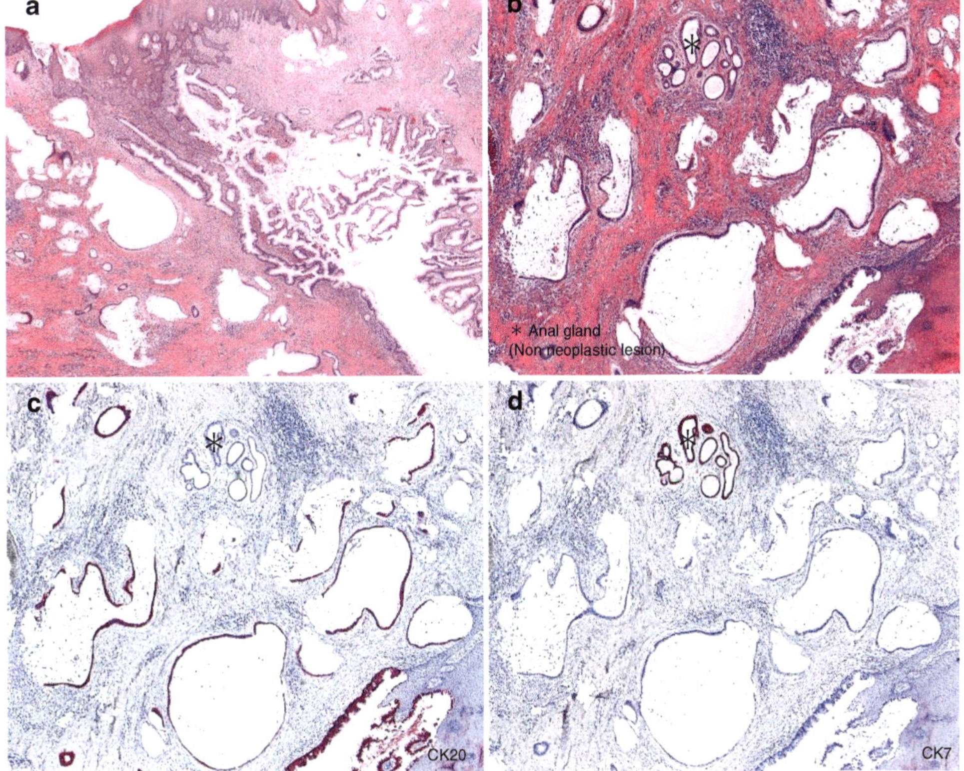

Fig. 68 H.E. and immunohistochemical staining: (**a** and **b**) The main lesion was a mucinous adenocarcinoma caused by a very well-differentiated tubular adenocarcinoma. (**c** and **d**) Immunohistochemically, the tumor was positive for cytokeratin (CK) 20 (**c**), but negative for CK7 (**d**), resembling adenocarcinoma of rectal type

The Pathological Diagnosis

- Anal canal and anus: Type 5, 50 × 40 mm, very well- to well-differentiated adenocarcinoma of the extramucosal type with extracellular mucous degeneration (mucinous adenocarcinoma), within the anorectal fistula (Figs. 66, 67, and 68), pT3, Ly0, V1a, BD1, INF b, Pn0, pPM0, pDM0, pRM0 pN0.
- Stage IIb (TNM): pT3, pN0, M0, P0, H0, R0, Cur A.

Summary

Adenocarcinoma has grown along the course of the fistula, suggesting that it originated from the fistula (Figs. 66 and 67). The tumor invaded beyond the conjoined longitudinal muscle of the anal canal and exceeded 5 cm in length, but the tumor volume was not large and there was no superficial exposure of the tumor except near the fistula opening. Histologically, the tumor was a very well-differentiated adenocarcinoma (Fig. 68), so it was not easy to diagnose the cancer clinically or pathologically. No lymph node metastasis was observed.

13 Case 18: Intramucosal Carcinoma of the Anal Canal Associated with Atypical Epithelium Around Reddish Polyp Lesions

Kitaro Futami and Hiroshi Tanabe

40s, male, type S, 20.2 years of illness

Onset in his 20s with ileus. Two years later, he underwent emergency surgery due to ileal perforation and was referred to our hospital under suspicion of Crohn's disease, where he was diagnosed and started medical therapy. Three years after the first surgery, he underwent a second intestinal resection procedure for complications of ileus. Eight years after the second surgery, he underwent endoscopic dilation for anastomotic stricture. Eleven years after the second surgery, he underwent a third intestinal resection procedure and was observed with immunomodulators. Four years later, the patient underwent regular colonoscopy and was diagnosed with a reddish polypoid lesion in the anal canal with atypical epithelium (Fig. 69). One month later, he underwent endoscopic resection and was diagnosed with well-differentiated adenocarcinoma (intramucosal carcinoma, Fig. 70), and a biopsy of the surrounding mucosa revealed atypical epithelium after endoscopic resection (Fig. 71). No abnormal findings were found on computed tomography or magnetic resonance imaging. CEA value: 3.5 ng/mL, CA19-9 value: 9.0 u/mL.

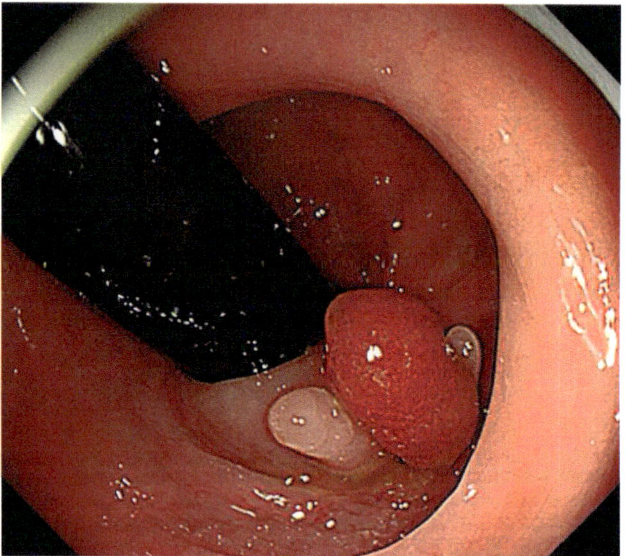

Fig. 69 Colonoscopy findings: A reddish polypoid lesion and atypical epithelium were detected

Surgery

Abdominoperineal resection, lymph node dissection, sigmoid colostomy

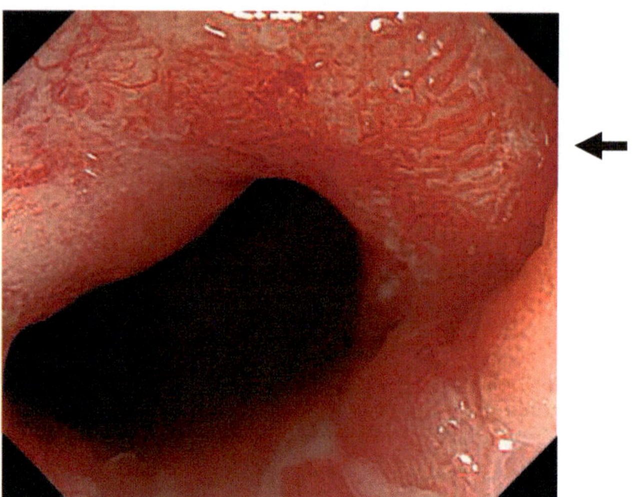

Fig. 70 Endoscope findings after endoscopic mucosal resection (EMR): An atypical epithelium was detected in the healed scar (arrow) of the anal canal

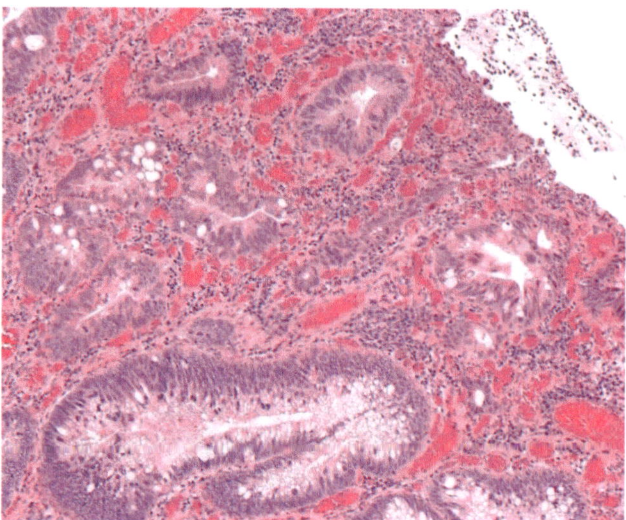

Fig. 71 Histology of the EMR specimen: EMR of an erythematous polyp of the anal canal showed a rectal-type well-differentiated tubular adenocarcinoma

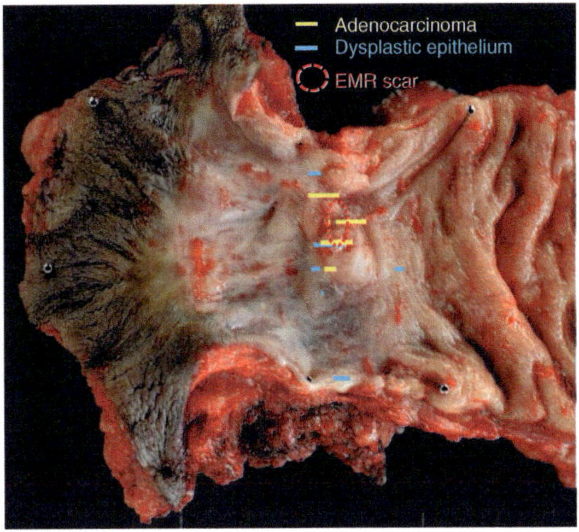

Fig. 72 Macroscopic findings of the resected specimen: Extension of adenocarcinoma was shown in yellow line and dysplastic epithelium was shown in blue line and scar of the EMR was shown in red circle

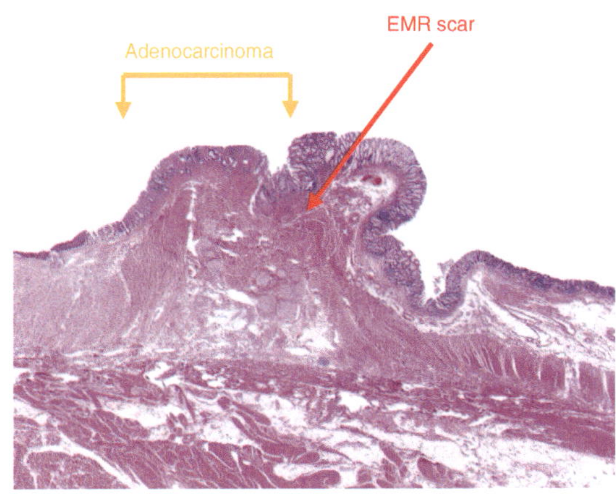

Fig. 73 Loupe finding: The surgical resection specimen showed an unevenly sized elevation on the Rb, and remnants of adenocarcinoma were found in the mucosa against the EMR scar background in the same area

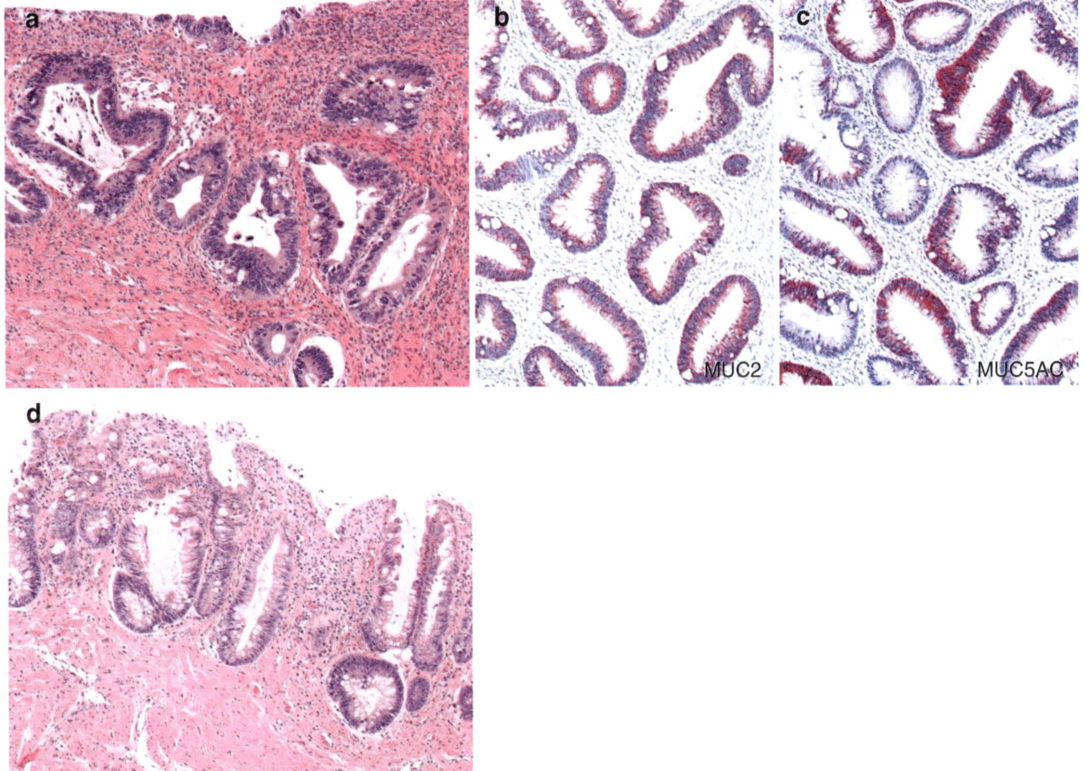

Fig. 74 H.E. and Immunohistochemical staining: (**a**) The tumor was well-differentiated tubular adenocarcinoma. (**b** and **c**) The tumor was immunohistochemically positive for both MUC2 (**b**) and MUC5AC (**c**), and the mucin phenotype of the carcinoma was mixed gastric and intestinal mucin phenotype. (**d**) Scattered dysplastic epithelium was detected

The Pathological Diagnosis

- Anal canal: Type 0-I+IIb, 15 × 10 mm, very well- to well-differentiated adenocarcinoma of rectal type (Figs. 72, 73, and 74a–c) with dysplastic epithelium (Fig. 74d) and healed ulcer, Ul-II to III, due to endoscopic mucosal resection, pTis (M), Ly0, V0, BD1, INF a, pPM0, pDM0, pN0. Stage 0: pTis, pN0, M0, P0, H0, R0, Cur A (Figs. 71, 72, 73, and 74)

Summary

This case prompted us to consider the indication for endoscopic mucosal resection of the anal region.

14 Case 19: Anal Cancer Diagnosed by a Transanal Biopsy Under Anesthesia Based on Increased Anal Pain and Elevated CEA Level

Kitaro Futami and Hiroshi Tanabe

50s, female, SL type, 31 years of illness

Onset in her teens with appendicitis. She was diagnosed by intraoperative findings and underwent ileocecal resection. Three bowel resection procedures and two anal surgeries for fistula were performed. Seventeen years after the onset, she developed an intra-abdominal abscess, so a fourth intestinal surgery was performed, and she was observed with medical therapies, including biologics, at the time of relapse. During this period, anal dilation, fistula drainage, and a biopsy of the anal canal mucosa were also performed for anorectal lesions. Eight years after the fourth surgery, the CEA level was elevated, and a biopsy under anesthesia was performed every 1–2 years for atypical epithelium. Very well-differentiated adenocarcinoma mixed with mucinous component was detected from the anal canal mucosa and anal fistula (Figs. 75 and 76). The cancer was detected as an irregular cystic mass lesion and suspected vaginal invasion on imaging examinations (Figs. 77 and 78).

Surgery

1. Posterior total pelvic exenteration, lymph node dissection, sigmoid colostomy;
2. Ileocolonic exclusion bypass for Crohn's disease.

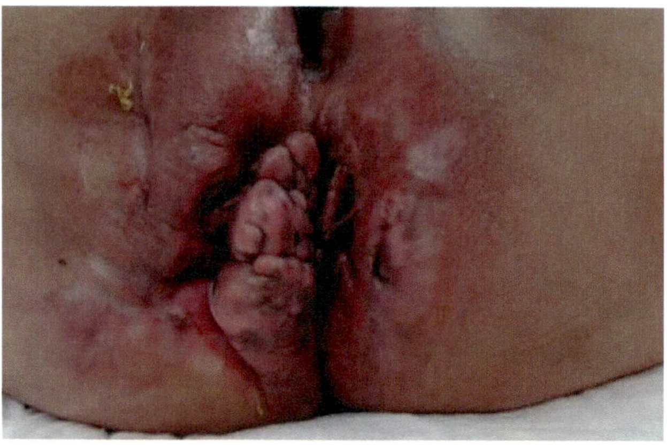

Fig. 75 Perianal findings: Complex anal lesions with circumferential fistula, thickened skin, and enlarged skin tags with anal stenosis

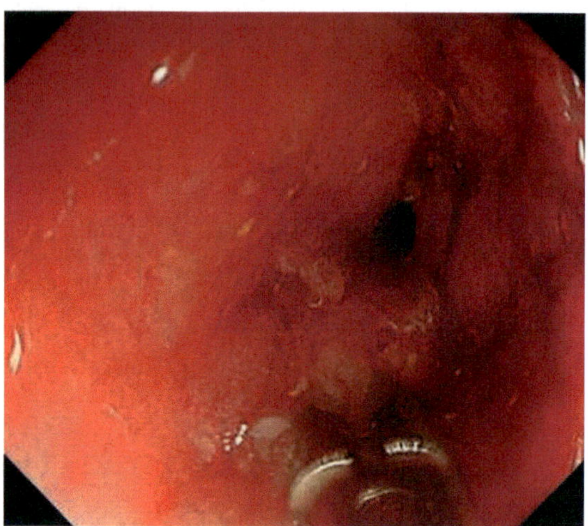

Fig. 76 Colonoscope findings: Poor observation by endoscopy due to severe stenosis, marked tenderness, and stenosis made outpatient endoscopy impossible

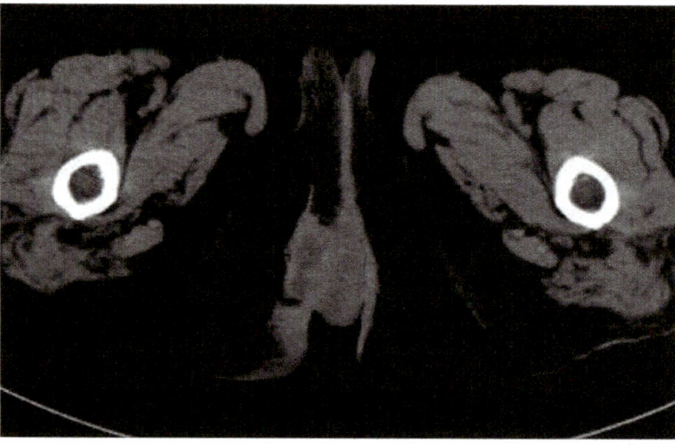

Fig. 77 CT findings: Cystic mass in the perianal region

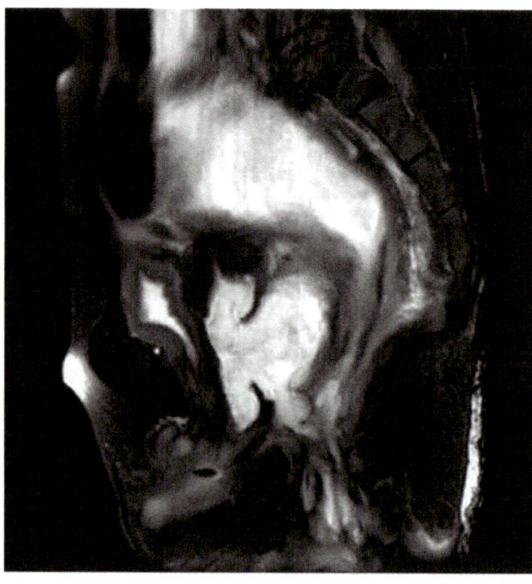

Fig. 78 MRI findings: Cystic mass with an unclear border to the vaginal septum (T2-weighted imaging)

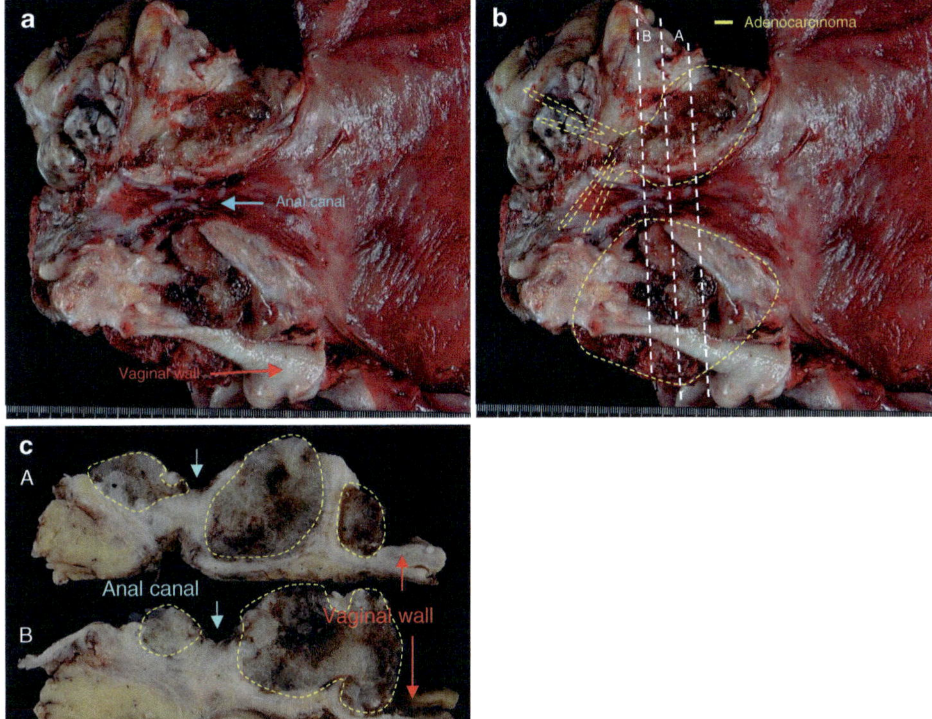

Fig. 79 Macroscopic finding of the resected specimen: (**a–c**). Carcinoma was located in the anal canal to the vaginal wall and carcinoma extension was schematically illustrated in yellow dotted line. It is presumed that the tumor grew and expanded to the lumen of the anal canal and vagina

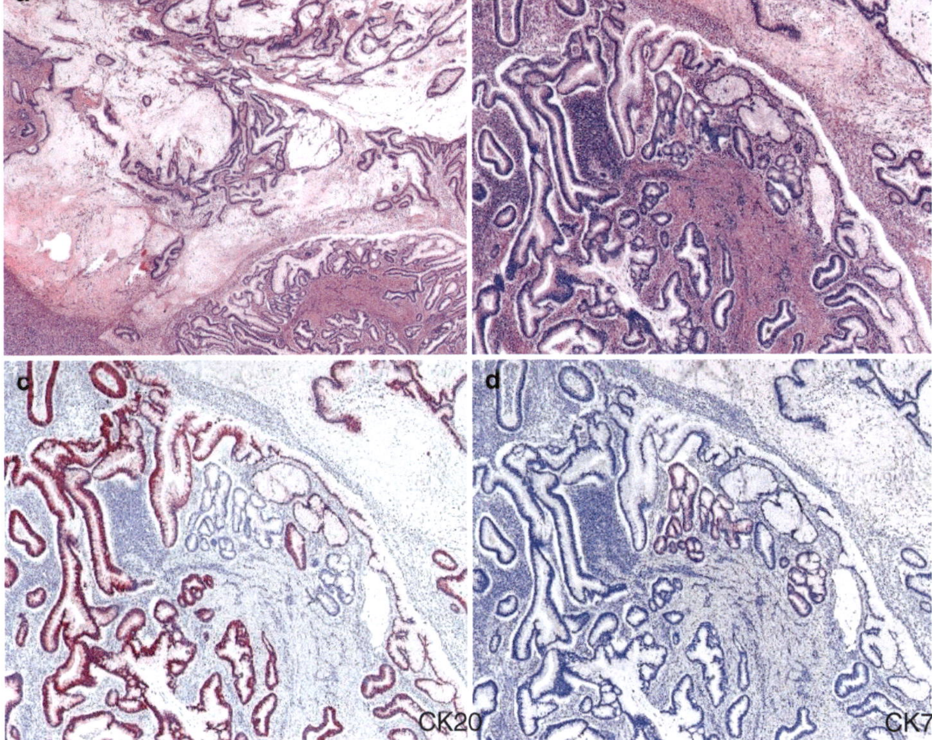

Fig. 80 H.E. and Immunohistochemical staining: (**a** and **b**) Mucinous carcinoma due to a well-differentiated adenocarcinoma was noted. (**c** and **d**) Immunohistochemically, most of the tumor glands were CK20-positive (**c**), and only a few were CK7-positive (**d**), resembling rectal-type adenocarcinoma

The Pathological Diagnosis

- Anal canal: Type 5, 90 mm, very well- to well-differentiated adenocarcinoma of extramucosal type with marked extracellular mucous degeneration (mucinous adenocarcinoma, Figs. 79 and 80), within anorectal-vaginal fistula, pT4 (vagina), Ly0, V1a, BD1, INF b, Pn0, pPM0, pDM0, pRM0, pN0.
- Stage IIIb (TNM): pT4, pN0, M0, P0, H0.

Summary

Mucinous adenocarcinoma was located at the anal canal to the vaginal wall (Figs. 79 and 80). The precise site of the lesion origin is unknown, but it is suggested that the tumor originated in the fistula.

Increasing anal pain is a risk factor for cancer invasion.

15 Case 20: Cancer of the Anus Diagnosed 2 Months After the Onset of Persistent Anal Pain

Kitaro Futami and Hiroshi Tanabe

40s, female, SL type, 26.9 years of illness

Onset in her teens with perianal surgery for fistula. She was diagnosed with CD. Eight years later, she started medical treatment. Previous abdominal surgeries were three bowel resection procedures and one cholecystectomy. For the anal lesions, seton drainage and anal dilation were performed. At the time of the final bowel surgery, there was neither pain nor sclerosis on palpation (Fig. 81). One year later, she visited the hospital complaining of anal pain that had persisted for 2 months (Fig. 82). Transanal and endoscopic examinations under anesthesia resulted in a cancer diagnosis: well- and poorly differentiated adenocarcinoma mixed with a mucinous component. The cancer was detected as an uneven solid mass lesion on MRI (Fig. 83). CEA value: 9.3 ng/mL, CA19-9 value: 1.0 u/mL.

Surgery

Abdominoperineal resection, lymph node dissection, resection of the posterior wall of the vagina, and sigmoid colostomy.

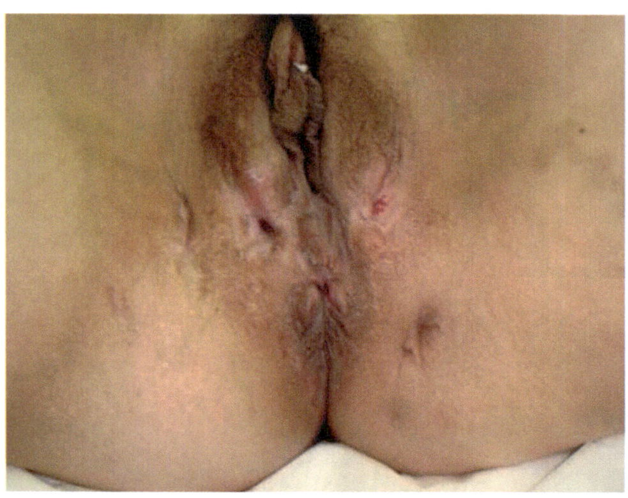

Fig. 81 Perianal findings 1 year earlier: No tenderness, no hardening, and no mass palpated

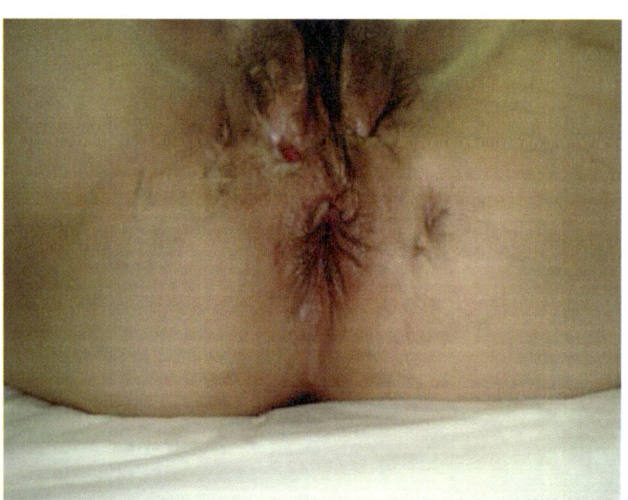

Fig. 82 Perianal findings at the time of the cancer diagnosis: A visual examination showed no change from 1 year earlier, but palpation showed significant sclerosis and tenderness in the surrounding area

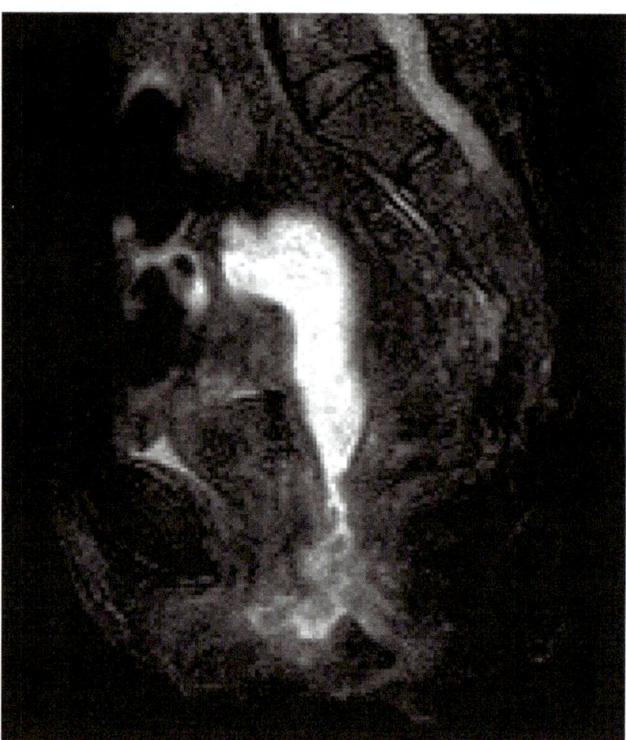

Fig. 83 MRI findings: Uneven solid mass with an unknown border and a high signal on T2-weighted imaging in the center of the anus

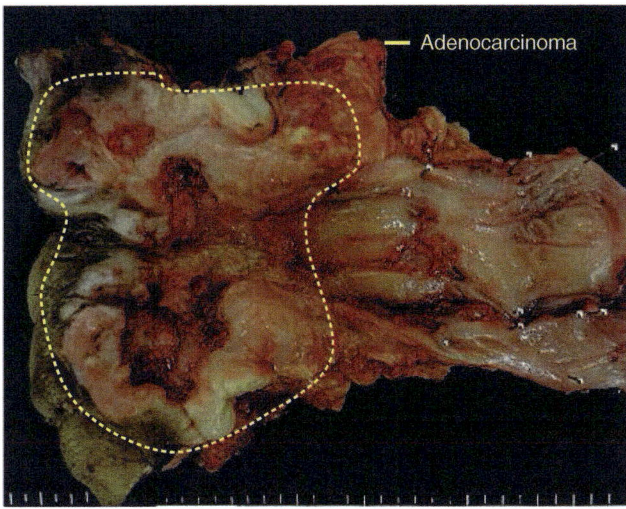

Fig. 84 Macroscopic findings of the resected specimen: Cancer extension was shown in yellow dotted lines. A circumferential type 5 advanced carcinoma extending from the anal canal to the rectum (Rb) was noted

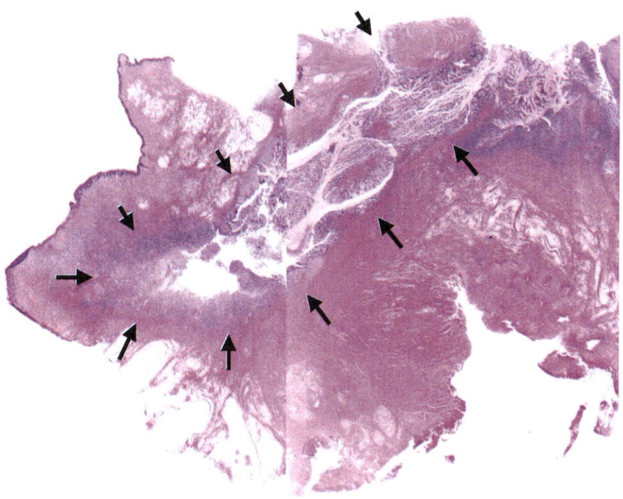

Fig. 86 Loupe finding: Growth and invasion of very well-differentiated adenocarcinoma was observed in the fistula

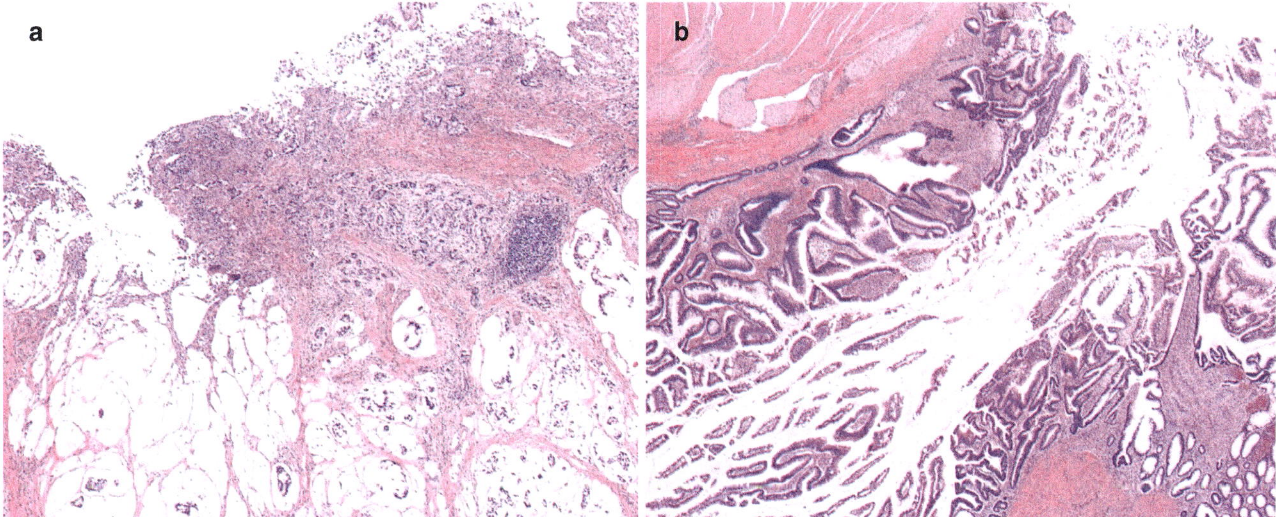

Fig. 85 H.E. staining: (**a** and **b**) The tumor was a mucinous carcinoma with a mixture of very well-differentiated rectal type (**b**) and poorly differentiated adenocarcinoma (**a**)

The Pathological Diagnosis

- Anal canal and rectum: Type 5, 100 mm, very well- to poorly differentiated adenocarcinoma of rectal type with marked intra- and extracellular mucous degeneration (mucinous adenocarcinoma) (Figs. 84, 85, and 86), pT4b (rt. vulva), Ly1c, V1a, INF c, Pn1b, pPM0, pDM0, pRM1, pN1b.
- Stage IIIc: pT4b, pN1b, M0, P0, H0, R1, Cur B.

Summary

A circumferential type 5 advanced mucinous adenocarcinoma extending from the anal canal to the rectum (Rb) was noted (Figs. 84, 85, and 86). Growth and invasion of very well-differentiated adenocarcinoma was observed in the fistula (Fig. 86). In the rectum (Rb), there was invasion up to the adventitia, and in the anal canal, there was an invasion from the external anal sphincter muscle to the right vulva, with marked vascular invasion but no lymph node metastasis.

The rapid-onset and persistent anal pain, in this case, led to the diagnosis.

GPSR Compliance

The European Union's (EU) General Product Safety Regulation (GPSR) is a set of rules that requires consumer products to be safe and our obligations to ensure this.

If you have any concerns about our products, you can contact us on ProductSafety@springernature.com

In case Publisher is established outside the EU, the EU authorized representative is:

Springer Nature Customer Service Center GmbH
Europaplatz 3
69115 Heidelberg, Germany

Batch number: 10371057

Printed by Printforce, the Netherlands